Praise for Wendell Potter and *Deadly Spin*

"As one former insurance executive testified before Congress, insurance companies are not only encouraged to find reasons to drop the seriously ill; they are rewarded for it. All of this is in service of meeting what [Potter] called 'Wall Street's relentless profit expectations.'"

—President Barack Obama, quoting Potter before Congress in September 2009

"A gripping indictment." **—Kate Pickert, *Time***

"Wendell Potter is a straight shooter—and he hits the bull's-eye here with an exposé of corporate power that reveals why real health care reform didn't happen, can't happen, and won't happen until that power is contained."

—Bill Moyers

"*Deadly Spin* makes clear what reporters were—and are—up against as they try, and often fail, to make the complex pros and cons of health care reform clear to citizens, as big-money players misdirect and obfuscate. More important, it illuminates what citizens are up against as they try to figure it out."

—Mike Hoyt, Executive Editor, *Columbia Journalism Review*

"Despite the damning revelations throughout his book, Mr. Potter's indictments of the industry he once served are far from heavy-handed; instead, they are suffused with the kind of transcendent empathy one finds in those who have undergone profound personal transformations . . . A tour de force . . . Eloquent."

—Pauline W. Chen, M.D., *New York Times*

"[Wendell Potter is] the Daniel Ellsberg of corporate America . . . People should read this book. The whole book lays it right out there about how the health insurance companies had bamboozled this country and lied, just outright lied about things." **—Michael Moore**

"The recently passed health care bill did many good things, including make health insurance available to more Americans and restrain some of the most egregious practices of the health insurance industry. It also forced more people to become customers of that industry. What the bill did *not* do is reform the health care system. Wendell Potter explains why not, and what went wrong."

—Howard Dean

"What sets this book apart is that it is one of the few volumes that examine ethical shortcomings of American public relations . . . This book is more than just one PR man's tell-all book about the insurance industry. It's a wake-up call."

—Gary Weiss, Portfolio.com

"[Potter] trenchantly critiques the failure of America's for-profit health-insurance system . . . [and his] street cred and deep knowledge of the industry make his indictment unusually vivid and compelling." **—*Publishers Weekly***

"Wendell Potter transformed the national debate over health care when he stood up and told the truth about the health insurance industry. By breaking the insurance industry's code of silence and explaining to his fellow Americans how health insurance companies put profits ahead of patient care, Wendell showed extraordinary courage. The compelling story of Wendell's conversion from a health care executive to an outspoken reform advocate is essential reading for anyone trying to understand the American health care system."

—Senator Jay Rockefeller of West Virginia

"Wendell Potter, former vice president of corporate communications with insurance giant CIGNA, now a fellow with the spin-busting Center for Media and Democracy, used media appearances and testimony before Congressional committees to expose the dark manipulations of fact that insurance firms use to preserve for-profit healthcare. Then he put it all on paper with a terrific book."

—*Nation*

"To get the country back on track, Potter exhorts consumers to adopt a healthy dose of skepticism toward corporate doublespeak. That's a sound prescription, one which no American can afford not to have filled."

—Joshua Kendall, *Boston Globe*

"Potter engagingly weaves together industry secrets with his own moral struggle and transformation into a whistleblower who tried to beat back the spin that nearly killed Obamacare." **—Emily Loftis, *Mother Jones***

"*Deadly Spin* is a must-read for all who want to learn more about what [the health reform law] is and what it is not. It is a handbook for social change."

—John Presta, *New York Journal of Books*

"Potter's *Deadly Spin* is an eye-opening account of the backroom antics of industries that do harm. You won't look at issues the same way after you read this book. If you can understand how "spin" works, you will be able to understand the money and tactics used to distort the truth. And we need to know the power propaganda has on us all." **—Kari Burns, *Chicago Life* magazine**

"In the end, the biggest contribution of *Deadly Spin* . . . is in how he uses his discussion of industry tactics to reframe the fundamental question about what kind of health care system we should have . . . Potter's broader theme is the threat of corporate power in America, and as we debate bank regulation and the freedom of corporations to make unrestricted political donations, this is certainly a hot issue in our country." **—Drew E. Altman, *Health Affairs***

"An illuminating, up-to-the-minute testimonial sure to garner widespread attention and controversy." **—*Kirkus Reviews***

"[Potter] ridicules the notion that America's free-market system can provide actual health care within a for-profit structure . . . This whistle-blower perspective will heighten discussion and debate on the vital topic of health care in America."

—Mary Whaley, *Booklist*

"The book's as dramatic and suspenseful as a good novel."

—Linda Greene, *Bloomington Alternative*

DEADLY SPIN

AN INSURANCE COMPANY INSIDER SPEAKS OUT ON HOW CORPORATE PR IS KILLING HEALTH CARE AND DECEIVING AMERICANS

Wendell Potter

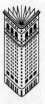

BLOOMSBURY PRESS

New York   Berlin   London   Sydney

Published by Bloomsbury Press, New York

All papers used by Bloomsbury Press are natural, recyclable products made
from wood grown in well-managed forests. The manufacturing processes
conform to the environmental regulations of the country of origin.

LIBRARY OF CONGRESS CATALOGING-IN-PUBLICATION DATA

Potter, Wendell, 1951–
Deadly spin : an insurance company insider speaks out on how corporate PR
is killing health care and deceiving Americans / Wendell Potter.—1st U.S. ed.
p. cm.
Other title: Insurance company insider speaks out on how
corporate PR is killing health care and deceiving Americans
Includes bibliographical references and index.
ISBN-13: 978-1-60819-281-6 (alk. paper)
ISBN-10: 1-60819-281-4 (alk. paper)
1. Health insurance—United States.   2. Insurance companies—Public
relations—United States.   I. Title.   II. Title: Insurance company insider speaks
out on how corporate PR is killing health care and deceiving Americans.
[DNLM: 1. Insurance, Health—economics—United States.   2. Delivery of Health
Care—economics—United States.   3. Health Care Reform—economics—United
States.   4. Health Care Sector—economics—United States.   5. Public Relations—
economics—United States. W 275 AA1 P825d 2010]

HG9383.P68 2010
659.2'936800973—dc22
201002270

First published by Bloomsbury Press in 2010
This paperback edition published in 2011

Paperback ISBN: 978-1-60819-404-9

1   3   5   7   9   10   8   6   4   2

Typeset by Westchester Book Group
Printed in the U.S.A. by Quad / Graphics, Fairfield, Pennsylvania

In memory of Barney DuBois, 1943–2011

*For Blaine and Pearl Potter. Thank you for the
many sacrifices you made for me and for leading
by example. I'm blessed to be your son.*

*For Alex and Emily. Thank you for putting up with an
often distant and cranky father while I was trying to find the
courage to do what I felt in my heart was the right thing.*

*And, especially, for Lou. Thank you for your patience and
steadfast support, for being the world's best mom and for
putting up with me, not only during my crisis of conscience
but since the day we met. You're the love of my life.*

Contents

Foreword to the Paperback Edition

On March 5, 2009, President Obama summoned health care leaders to the White House to start talking about reforming our health care system. At that meeting, Karen Ignagni, the health insurance industry's top lobbyist, looked the president in the eye and said the industry was "committed" to health care reform. She said, "We want to work with you. We want to work with the members of Congress on a bipartisan basis here. You have our commitment. We hear the American people about what's not working. We've taken that seriously. You have our commitment to play, to contribute, and to help pass health care reform this year."

A few months later, a soft-spoken former health insurance industry executive named Wendell Potter came to the United States Senate Committee on Commerce, Science, and Transportation, where I serve as chairman, and warned us not to believe a word Ignagni said. In the compelling testimony he gave before my committee on June 24, 2009, Wendell told me and my fellow senators that we had "good reason to question the honesty and trustworthiness of the insurance industry." Ignore the industry's cynical charm offensive, he urged us, and focus instead on how health insurance companies make money at the expense of their patients.

In his testimony that day and every day since, Wendell Potter has been telling anyone who will listen about how for-profit health insurance companies really work. In his calm, unflappable style, Wendell recalls his direct experiences as a health insurance executive and explains that health insurance companies are driven more by profits than by patient care; that they worry little about keeping people healthy, and a great deal about their next quarterly conference call with Wall Street analysts.

Thanks to Wendell, we learned the insider's health industry jargon that you will never hear during their carefully scripted public relations campaigns. He told us about "purging," where insurance companies use large price increases to force small businesses with sick workers to drop their policies. He described how insurers push employers to go "full replacement," or move employees from major medical coverage to plans that force them to pay for more of their health care out of their own pockets.

Wendell also explained how insurance companies relentlessly focus on an obscure financial indicator known as the "medical-loss ratio," (MLR). In the upside-down world of for-profit health insurance, providing more health care to patients is viewed as a "loss."

"I could always tell how busy my day was going to be when CIGNA announced earnings by looking at the MLR numbers," Wendell writes. If the company had reduced its medical spending from the last quarter, Wall Street investors were happy and stock prices rose. But even small increases in medical spending could trigger dropping stock prices and sell-offs. On these days, Wendell says, "my phone would ring constantly with financial reporters wanting to know what was wrong."

As a trained journalist and experienced public relations executive, Wendell knew how to handle these calls. He knew how to tell a good story and give a reporter a pithy quote. Even more important, he knew how to keep his cool when the health insurance industry came under attack.

Ironically, these are the very same skills that have made Wendell one of the most credible and persuasive critics of the health insurance industry in our country today. Wendell didn't appear at the Senate Commerce Committee in June of 2009 because he had an ax to grind or scores to settle. In fact, Wendell goes out of his way to express admiration for his former colleagues in the health insurance industry. Wendell decided to speak out because at a time when serious debate was under way about how to fix our ailing health care system, he knew how the health insurance industry really worked, and he felt a moral obligation to share what he knew with the rest of us.

Wendell's public appearance before my committee that day was an act of personal courage. Wendell talks very candidly in this book about the sophisticated, under-the-radar smear campaigns health insurance companies orchestrate against their opponents. He fully expected to be on the receiving end of one of these attacks.

But curiously, Wendell's former colleagues in the industry have never tried to discredit or refute him. Instead, his former colleagues "decided that the best way to deal with me was to pretend I didn't exist." Quite simply, an industry that spends tens of millions of dollars every year countering negative publicity and shaping public opinion has still not yet figured out how to rebut one man telling the truth about how for-profit health care really works.

Wendell is such a genuinely humble person that I don't know whether he appreciates the key role his testimony played in the debates that preceded the passage of the health care reform law. His testimony made it impossible for policymakers to pretend that we did not need a lot more accountability and transparency in the health insurance industry if we were going to fix the system for the American people.

The health care reform law that Congress passed in March 2010 made important progress on a number of problems Wendell identified. The law has forced health insurance companies to disclose a lot more information about their business practices, it has stopped companies from cutting off people after they get sick, and it turned those medical-loss ratios Wendell told us about into a tool that measures whether consumers are getting a good value for their premium dollars.

For the first time in a hundred years, we're making real progress on some of the most difficult and important public policy issues our nation has ever faced. Yes, we are making some adjustments to the health care reform law along the way, but we are moving forward as never before. Over the next few years, millions of our fellow citizens will have access to affordable, high-quality health care for the first time.

Anyone who reads Wendell Potter's inside account of how the health insurance industry worked in the years before health care reform will gain a clearer picture of the powerful forces at play in our health care system, and will understand why the health care reform law was needed to protect consumers. Wendell's story is a stark reminder of why going back to "business as usual" in our health care system is not an option.

Senator John D. Rockefeller IV
May 2011

Foreword

When my old friend and colleague Wendell Potter contacted me in 2008, it was the first time I'd heard from him in years. He told me he'd quit his job as head of corporate communications at the health insurer CIGNA and was trying to decide what to do next. I remember asking him what had happened at CIGNA to make him leave, and he said it was a "long story" but that he'd tell me sometime. The short version, he said then, was that he had decided to come back to the "real world."

In many ways, I've learned subsequently, it was Wendell who had been living in the real world—where corporate greed and human indifference are the daily norm. It was the rest of us, including me, who were living the fantasy, thinking that America's free-market system could provide actual health care for its people through a for-profit structure.

I've known Wendell since the late spring of 1973, when he came to the old *Memphis Press-Scimitar* as a summer intern after graduating from the University of Tennessee in Knoxville. I was the rewrite man and an assistant city editor at the now defunct afternoon daily, which meant I was the one who handled the rough copy that came from reporters and interns, frequently with deadlines staring us in the face. Wendell made his mark quickly.

He knew the right questions to ask, and he knew how to get the answers and put them into words. His copy may have needed a little tweaking from time to time, but he was a quick learner, even thanking me for some of the changes I made. (How rare is that?) Everyone on the city desk quickly knew we had a keeper, and Wendell rose rapidly through the journalistic ranks at Scripps Howard in the next few years—eventually winding up as the youngest reporter the chain ever assigned to cover Washington, D.C., politics.

As Wendell and I chatted in the months after reconnecting in 2008, it became evident that he had an even bigger story to tell. We even talked about him writing a book, but he was still unsure about what he would do next, actually reveling in the first taste of anonymity he'd experienced in decades.

But things changed. Health care reform became front-page news. Wendell recognized that the PR barrage unleashed by his former industry was skewing the debate on this vital issue. He decided to speak out, regardless of the consequences. The result was months of public appearances—in person, on TV, and in congressional hearings—and now he's finally written that book. You're holding it.

Deadly Spin is a revelation about America's health care system unlike anything else you've seen. There are a lot of books and articles about health care reform, but none of them provide the insider's perspective like this one.

As an old newshound, I'm a little cynical about anything I read. And you should be, too. I ask myself, who's telling me this and why? To me, the chapters that follow are the work of a first-rate investigative reporter who spent twenty years on his undercover assignment. No one actually gave him the assignment, and he wasn't even aware he was on one—until the events occurred that he outlines for us in the book. But once a journalist, always a journalist.

We're fortunate to have Wendell Potter back on the beat.

Barney DuBois
Memphis, Tennessee
July 2010

Introduction

*The twentieth century has been characterized by three developments
of great political importance: the growth of democracy, the growth of
corporate power, and the growth of corporate propaganda as a means
of protecting corporate power against democracy.*

—ALEX CAREY[1]

*You have our commitment to play, to contribute, and to help pass
health care reform this year.*

—KAREN IGNAGNI[2]

ABOUT forty-five thousand people die in America every year
because they have no health insurance.[3]

I am partly responsible for some of the deaths making up that
shameful statistic.

As a senior public relations executive, or "spinmeister," for two
decades with two of the largest for-profit health insurance companies
in the United States—Humana and CIGNA—it was my job to enhance those firms' reputations. But as one of the industry's top public
relations executives and media spokesmen, I also helped create and

perpetuate myths that had no other purpose but to sustain those companies' extraordinarily high profitability.

For example, if you are among those who believe that the United States has "the best health care system in the world" despite overwhelming evidence to the contrary—it's because my fellow spinmeisters and I succeeded brilliantly at what we were paid very well to do with your premium dollars. In fact, the United States ranks 47th in life expectancy at birth, behind Bosnia, and 54th, behind Bangladesh, in "fairness," a measure of the extent to which the best care is available equally throughout a country.

And if you were persuaded that the health care reform bill President Barack Obama signed into law in March 2010 was "a government takeover of the health care system," my former colleagues and I earned every penny of our handsome salaries. Not to mention our bonuses.

From the first day of the Clinton administration in 1993 until shortly before the election of Obama, I was a behind-the-scenes leader in every industry effort to kill any reform legislation that threatened insurance company profits. Although I told people during that period that I never lied to a reporter, the reality is that I often did—but in such subtle ways that I could never even acknowledge to myself that I was purposely trying to mislead. At the time, I was unaware that I was feeding the media and the public false information, and so caught up in the industry's swirling spin machine that I was oblivious to it.

Had it not been for a series of events that occurred in 2007—events that, as someone raised as a Southern Baptist, I can't help believing were part of some kind of divine intervention—I would probably still be spinning for health insurers.

In retrospect, it seems as if it were predestined that I would become either a witness to or a participant in those events, which would reveal to me just how corrupt and deadly the American health insurance industry had become, and also how far I had strayed from my own moral path. By the end of 2007, it was inevitable that I would leave my job and begin speaking out against what I consider now to be an evil system built and sustained on greed.

I don't mean to imply that all people who work for health insurance companies are greedier or more evil than other Americans. In fact, many of them feel—and justifiably so—that they are helping millions of people get the care they need. Mostly, they are just as unaware as I was for much of my career of what really motivates the top executive officers of the companies they work for.

The health insurance industry today is dominated by a cartel of large, for-profit corporations. By necessity and by law, the top priority of the officers of these companies is to "enhance shareholder value." When that's your top priority, you are motivated more by the obligation to meet Wall Street's relentless profit expectations than by the obligation to meet the medical needs of your policyholders. Some nonprofit insurers still operate in the United States, but they are now behaving the same way—as they must, in order to compete with their for-profit counterparts, lest they be forced to put themselves up for sale or close, as many have already done.

It was not until late in my career that I became aware of the lengths to which insurance company executives will go to meet Wall Street's expectations. The further up the corporate ladder I climbed, the more I saw, and the more disillusioned I became with my job, my profession, and my industry.

As it played out, my full awakening occurred during the events I alluded to above, during the last eight months of 2007. I was involved in three episodes that opened my eyes to how unscrupulous my industry had become and how it failed sick and suffering Americans every day. I will describe all three of these events and their significance— not only to me but to the state of the U.S. health care system and to the future of our democracy—in the following chapters.

I will also attempt to explain why it is vital to understand the role of the public relations industry—the spin machine—in our public discourse and in our lives, how to recognize it, and what we can do about it.

More than half a century ago, Vance Packard revealed in his book *The Hidden Persuaders* how advertisers use subliminal tactics and other psychological techniques to get people to buy certain products and to vote for certain political candidates. Packard described his book as "an attempt to explore a strange and rather exotic new area" of American life.

"It is about the large-scale efforts being made, often with impressive success, to channel our unthinking habits, our purchasing decisions, and our thought processes by the use of insights gleaned from psychiatry and the social sciences," he wrote. "Typically these efforts take place beneath our level of awareness; so that the appeals which move us are often, in a sense, 'hidden.' The result is that many of us are being influenced and manipulated, far more than we realize, in the patterns of our everyday lives."[4]

Americans are probably more aware of the techniques advertisers use to influence decisions today than they were fifty years ago. But comparatively few are aware of the more insidious techniques used by PR professionals to manipulate public opinion and, consequently, public policy. What I hope to accomplish in this book is to pull the curtain back to reveal the techniques employed by practitioners of the dark arts of PR—from the use of "third-party advocates" to the creation of front groups, from the staging of PR "charm offensives" to the selective disclosure of information and misinformation—which influence people's thoughts and actions in ways that advertising cannot. In that sense, this book is as much about PR as it is about health care. Deceptive practices corrupt public debate and policy in many industries, but health care offers a timely and particularly egregious example, which I can attest to firsthand.

If advertisers are the hidden persuaders, PR practitioners are the "invisible persuaders," to borrow the term British author David Michie used in the title of his 1998 book about the growing influence of unseen PR advisers in the United Kingdom.[5]

PR people do not create ads that can be seen or heard or touched.

They create perceptions without any public disclosure of who is doing the persuading or for what purposes.

Although PR techniques remain a mystery to most people, the art of invisible persuasion has long been in the making. PR and corporate propaganda go back to the early part of the twentieth century. One of the first practitioners was Ivy Lee—often called the father of modern PR—who was hired by the Standard Oil Company to transform John D. Rockefeller Jr.'s reputation from "biggest criminal of all time," as his detractors called him, to "the great benefactor of society," as he is more commonly known today. Lee's biggest competitor at the time was Edward Bernays, who was able to persuade young women to start smoking cigarettes on behalf of his client, the American Tobacco Company.

From such precedents grew a profession reaching from big tobacco to the military-industrial complex, and now to health care. It uses deceptive tactics to influence how the public thinks and, ultimately, how lawmakers vote. Over the last several decades, through the skillful use of such tactics, the American health insurance industry has created a perception of its role and usefulness—its raison d'être—that obscures its real goal: profits.

Many of the biggest and most influential PR firms in the country, including APCO Worldwide and Porter Novelli, have carried out deception-based campaigns over many years for health insurers, as I will describe. Their attitude and approach have all too often been to do whatever it takes to win. I should know; I often hired them for just this reason.

That said, it is not my intention to write a book that condemns an entire profession. Many—probably most—PR professionals follow guidelines established years ago by the Public Relations Society of America, an organization that encourages ethical behavior among its members and all PR practitioners, and of which I have been a proud member for more than three decades. In fact, PRSA was one of the first organizations—and there have been many—to invite me to speak to its membership to explain why I had become such an outspoken critic of both the health insurance industry and the PR profession.

PRSA also published my comments on professional conduct in a recent edition of its quarterly magazine, the *Public Relations Strategist*. In that interview, I noted that PR people who veer off the ethical path, as I did, are often those who work for publicly traded companies—which most large insurers now are—that are under constant pressure from investors to meet profit expectations.

It was this same pressure, I know for a fact, that led otherwise-decent men and women to plan and implement the fearmongering, deception-based PR campaign to erode public support during the recent health care reform debate. Their orchestrated attacks during the debate eventually made it politically unfeasible for Congress to pass the kind of radical health care reform desired by President Obama and many American voters—and that Democratic leaders just months earlier had believed could be enacted.

Many health care reform advocates naïvely thought that with Obama in the White House and Democrats in control of Congress—and with the health insurance industry claiming to be on the side of the angels this time—the stars had finally aligned for comprehensive health care reform that would lead, with the stroke of the president's pen, to universal coverage. They thought that achieving the goal of every Democratic president since Franklin Roosevelt—which every other developed country on the planet had achieved years ago—was all but inevitable.

It was because of that misplaced confidence, based to no small extent on the health insurance industry's PR offensive, that I decided I had to speak out.

I warned members of Congress—in a series of appearances before House and Senate committees—that if the bill Congress ultimately passed included many of the so-called solutions insurers were "bringing to the table," and if it did not include a public insurance option to compete with private insurers, it might as well be called the "Health Insurance Industry Profit Protection and Enhancement Act."

The bill the president signed will indeed protect and enhance the health insurance industry's profits for many years to come. It will also do a lot of good for a lot of people. Among other things, it will expand the Medicaid program to cover many more low-income families; it will make it illegal for insurance companies to deny coverage because of preexisting conditions; it will provide tax credits to small businesses to encourage them to offer health benefits to their employees; and it will close the infamous gap in the Medicare drug benefit known as the "doughnut hole."

But in many other significant ways, the industry's spin worked as intended. The new law does *not* include the public option the president once said was essential "to keep insurance companies honest"— and it *does* include a provision that candidate Obama was adamantly opposed to: a mandate that all Americans not eligible for an existing public program buy coverage from a private insurer. Candidate Obama said during the campaign that he did not think people should be forced to buy insurance they could not afford. The insurance industry and many members of Congress persuaded President Obama to change his mind. As a result, insurers will get billions of dollars in new revenues from people required by law to buy their products and billions more from the government to subsidize premiums for people who can't afford them. Because of the way the legislation came together on Capitol Hill, the complex bill that reached the president's desk would not really work without the so-called individual mandate.

While there are several new regulations that insurers will have to abide by—or seek to weaken or overturn in the months and years ahead—they got much of what they wanted and were able to eliminate most of what they didn't like.

Despite the insurance industry's successes and my disappointments with the final bill, I did not join the many progressives who were following the Republican lead in urging Congress to scrap it and start over.

My support of the bill led a few on the far left to call me a "corporatist" and a double agent for the insurance industry. I hope this book will explain—by putting the recent debate in historical perspective and by providing a behind-the-scenes look at how the advocates for reform were often out-maneuvered and out-"messaged"—why scrapping the bill, despite its flaws, would have been the worst thing Congress could have done. Had the legislation failed, the industry and its political allies would have been further emboldened, and neither Congress nor any future president would have taken the political risk of attempting meaningful reform for years, as was the case after the Clinton plan failed. The perception of health care reform as the untouchable "third rail of American politics" would have been solidified.

This book will also explain why the enactment of the Patient Protection and Affordable Care Act of 2010 is only the first halting step in the direction we need to keep moving in to make the U.S. health care system better, in terms of quality of care, cost efficiency, and equitability. It will detail some of the serious problems that lawmakers must tackle next—and soon. It will describe the disturbing trends in health insurance—which the new law only partially addresses—that are pushing more Americans into the ranks of the *under*insured. It will explain how a law enacted almost thirty years ago to protect employee pension benefits has made it nearly impossible for 130 million Americans now enrolled in employer-sponsored health insurance plans to seek relief from the courts when their insurance companies deny coverage—and why many of the provisions of the new law will not apply to them. It will also chronicle the ascendancy of corporate PR in general at a time when the mainstream media is in decline and the Supreme Court has given corporations the freedom they have long sought to spend unlimited amounts of money to influence elections and, as a result, public policy.

Finally, this book will describe what the latter trends mean not only for our health care system but also for our democracy and way of life—and explain why we will continue down a fast track to losing both unless we start paying attention to these trends.

In conclusion, I will suggest ways we can fight back.

For I believe that unless we do fight back—and with urgency—the twenty-first century will be dominated by the retrenchment of democracy and the unbridled growth of corporate power, enabled by increasingly unchallenged propaganda.

CHAPTER I

The Beginning

M Y name is Wendell Potter and for twenty years, I worked as a senior executive at health insurance companies, and I saw how they confuse their customers and dump the sick—all so they can satisfy their Wall Street investors."

That is how I introduced myself to the U.S. Senate Commerce, Science, and Transportation Committee on June 24, 2009. The committee's chair, Senator Jay Rockefeller (D-W. Va.), had asked me to testify as part of his investigation into health insurance company practices that for years had been swelling the ranks of the uninsured and the underinsured in the United States.

I explained how insurance companies make promises they have no intention of keeping, how they flout regulations designed to protect consumers, and how they make it nearly impossible to understand—or even obtain—information needed by consumers. I described how for-profit insurance companies, in their constant quest to meet Wall Street's profit expectations, routinely cancel the coverage of policyholders who get sick, and how they "purge" small businesses when their employees' medical claims exceed what underwriters expected.

I knew that as soon as I said those words my life would change forever. It did—but in ways I never could have imagined.

I had quit my job as head of public relations at CIGNA—a job that had paid me deep into six figures—because I could no longer serve in good conscience as a spokesman for an industry whose routine practices amount to a death sentence for thousands of Americans every year.

I did not intend to go public as a critic of the industry. But it gradually became clear to me that the industry's duplicitous PR strategy was going to manipulate public opinion and likely shape health care reform in ways that would benefit insurance company executives and their Wall Street masters far more than most other Americans.

I was eventually compelled to pull back the curtain on the industry's deception-based PR strategy, which comprised two active fronts. One was a highly visible "charm offensive" designed to create an image of the industry as an advocate of reform—and a good-faith partner with the president and Congress in achieving it. The second front was a secret, fearmongering campaign using front groups and business and political allies as shills to disseminate misinformation and lies, with the sole intent of killing any reform that might hinder profits.

I had left my job at CIGNA in May 2008, but it wasn't until ten months later that I realized I couldn't stay on the sidelines. As it turned out, it would be a fellow Tennessean who gave me one of the final shoves off the sidelines and into the spotlight and the new role of whistle-blower, as many people have called me.

It was March 5, 2009, and I was channel surfing for some news about the health care reform summit that President Obama was holding at the White House that day. Of the 120 or so people at the summit, many were from special interests that had the largest stakes financially in a reformed health care system: doctors, hospitals, drug and medical-device manufacturers, and, of course, insurers. Knowing that these groups had played a lead role in killing Bill and Hillary Clinton's reform plan fifteen years earlier, Obama wanted to keep them from doing the same this time around. Having campaigned as someone who could bring people with diverse points of view together to work toward the common good, Obama had brought the top lobbyists of each special interest group to his kickoff reform "table"—which the Clintons had not done—and openly solicited the groups' support and cooperation. To win their support, his administration would eventually cut side deals with some of them, most notably the drugmakers.

I flipped to MSNBC just as Tamron Hall was getting ready to interview Republican representative Zach Wamp, from Tennessee's Third Congressional District. I'm also from east Tennessee, although I have lived in Philadelphia since CIGNA relocated me to the company's headquarters there in 1997. I grew up in Mountain City and Kingsport, both in the northeastern part of the state near the Virginia line. Wamp lives in Chattanooga, in the southeastern part of the state near the Georgia line.

When Hall asked Wamp about his views on the president's ideas for reform, he just about called Obama a Marxist: "It's probably the next major step towards socialism. I hate to sound so harsh, but . . . this literally is a fast march towards socialism, where the government is bigger than the private sector in our country, and health care's the next major step, so we oughta all be worried about it."

He then started accusing the Democrats of wanting to redistribute wealth in the country by taking money away from those who already had health care to pay for those who didn't have it, many of whom, in his view, were just irresponsible bums waiting for a handout.

"Listen," he said. "The forty-five million people that don't have health insurance—about half of them choose not to have health insurance. Half of 'em don't have any choice, but half of 'em choose to, what's called 'go naked,' and just take a risk of getting sick. They end up in the emergency room, costing you and me a whole lot more money. How many illegal immigrants are in this country today, getting our health care? Gobs of 'em!"

As I listened to Wamp's rant, I knew exactly where he'd gotten his talking points: from me.

He was using the same misleading, intentionally provocative, and xenophobic talking points that I had helped write while serving on the Strategic Communications Advisory Committee of the insurers' biggest trade group, America's Health Insurance Plans (AHIP). We PR types had created those talking points, with help from language and polling experts, and given them to the industry's lobbyists with instructions to get them into the hands of every "friendly" member of Congress. Most of the friendly ones were Republicans, and most were friendly because they had received a lot of money over the years in campaign contributions from insurance company executives and their political action committees.

(In spirited remarks on the House floor shortly before the vote on final reform legislation in 2010, Representative Anthony Weiner [D-N.Y.] called the Republican Party a "wholly owned subsidiary of the insurance industry." As someone who had managed CIGNA's PAC contributions for several years, I knew Weiner's remark had the ring of truth. CIGNA and other big insurers have contributed considerably more to Republicans than to Democrats.)

I was dismayed to hear Wamp's demagogic remarks—and not just because I'd had a hand in writing his script, but also because I know his district well. If anybody in America could benefit from the Democrats' vision of reform, it would be those who live in the counties he represents. Many are rural and remote, with high percentages of people who are either uninsured or underinsured. The per capita and household incomes in most of his counties are far below the national average. Yet the Third District's representative—contrary to the best interests of his constituents—was saying exactly what the insurance industry wanted him to say.

Later that evening, I saw a couple of TV reports about the summit. One of the clips featured Karen Ignagni, AHIP's president, standing up at the summit and telling the president he could count on her and the health insurance industry.

"Thank you, Mr. President," she said. "Thank you for inviting us

to participate in this forum. I think, on behalf of our entire membership, they would want to be able to say to you this afternoon and
everyone here that we understand we have to earn a seat at this table.
We've already offered a comprehensive series of proposals. We want to
work with you. We want to work with the members of Congress on a
bipartisan basis here. You have our commitment. We hear the American people about what's not working. We've taken that seriously."

Turning in one of her best performances to date, she added, "You
have our commitment to play, to contribute, and to help pass health
care reform this year."

The president—having just been played like a Stradivarius by
one of the best lobbyists ever to hit Washington—said, "Good. Thank
you, Karen. That's good news. That's America's Health Insurance
Plans."

The crowd cheered and applauded. They all seemed to be buying
it—but I wasn't, not by a long shot. I wasn't surprised, either, at the
president's and the crowd's reactions to what she had said.

Ignagni is one of the most effective communicators and—with a
salary and bonuses of $1.94 million in 2008—one of the highest-paid
special interest advocates in Washington. I've known her since she left
the AFL-CIO in the early 1990s to lead one of AHIP's predecessors,
the Group Health Association of America, an HMO trade group of
which Humana was a member when I worked for that insurer. I knew
from the first time I met her that she was the perfect choice to lead the
insurance industry. She is smart, telegenic, articulate, charming, a
strong leader, and a brilliant strategist. Following her success in shaping
to her industry's liking the legislation creating the Medicare prescription drug program, Princeton economist Uwe Reinhardt commented,
"Whatever AHIP pays her is not enough."

I realized after watching the exchange between Ignagni and
Obama that I had seen both sides of the industry's duplicitous PR
campaign in a single day. Ignagni was saying what she knew the president and the inside-the-Beltway crowd wanted to hear, while Wamp

was saying what the industry wanted him to say to the rest of the world. He was a tool in the industry's effort to use "third parties" to kill key elements of the president's plan, if not all of it, by scaring and lying to the public.

But it was another televised interview the following Monday that pushed me from the sidelines and into the fray. Four days after the White House summit, Chris Matthews was interviewing Mike Tuffin, AHIP's executive vice president of strategic communications, on his MSNBC show, *Hardball*. "The same people who helped kill the Clintons' efforts back in the '90s are on the other side now," Matthews said in introducing Tuffin. "Times have changed. The worm has turned. The cosmos has shifted. Some of the bad guys are becoming perhaps the good guys."

There was no doubt about it: Tuffin was on the show as part of AHIP's charm offensive.

"This time," he told Matthews, "we're coming to the table with solutions. We want to be part of the process. We pledged that to the president. We're calling for new regulations on our industry to make sure everyone has guaranteed access to coverage." He thus joined Ignagni in spinning the fiction that, for the first time ever, insurers were willing to accept more regulations and change their ways so that everybody in America could "have access to affordable, quality care" (a favorite term of industry leaders).

And just like Obama, Matthews seemed to be falling for it.

THE TIME HAD COME TO MAKE A MOVE

I realized that with both political leaders and the media buying the industry line, ordinary Americans had little chance of understanding what was happening. Health care reform was about to be eviscerated, again. I couldn't sit back and watch this happen. I immediately began making phone calls to people I thought might help me connect with organizations advocating for *real* reform. My first thought was that I could be an anonymous adviser who could help them expose the industry's dirty tricks. I wasn't yet sure I wanted to play a visible role at that point. I was afraid the industry would retaliate in some way.

To explain why I changed my mind and decided to go public as a critic of the industry, I need to explain where I came from and how I wound up being an insurance company flack in the first place.

I was born in Banner Elk, North Carolina, on July 16, 1951, not because my parents lived there but because they didn't have access to "affordable, quality care" in the tiny town where they did live, on the other side of the Blue Ridge Mountains—Mountain City, Tennessee. There was no hospital in Mountain City, or the entire county for that matter. My parents, Blaine and Pearl Potter, were born and raised in Johnson County—Mountain City is the county seat—one of the most beautiful places on earth, in my opinion, but where, even today, it is hard to make a living. There were only two doctors in all of Johnson County when I was born. Mom didn't want either of them to have anything to do with bringing me into this world. She had heard good things about the hospital in Banner Elk, so that's where Dad drove her, over thirty miles of winding, mountainous roads, when she went into labor.

Affordable, quality health care wasn't the only thing my folks didn't have easy access to. Money was another. I've never met a smarter, harder-working, and more resourceful man than my dad, but I probably earned more in one year at CIGNA than he earned in the twenty-some years he worked in a brutally hot factory before retiring in 1980. Before his factory job, when I was born, he and Mom had a small farm (the main money crop was tobacco) and ran a little country store, Potter's Grocery, on Spear Branch Road in Mountain City. Dad built both the store and our first house, next door to it, with help from a couple of my uncles. Like most of the houses on Spear Branch Road at the time, ours did not have an indoor bathroom. We would not have one, in fact, until we moved when I was six to what seemed to me a huge city, Kingsport, about fifty miles to the west.

For more than a year before we moved to Kingsport, Dad "commuted" to the Blue Ridge glass plant, where a relative had been able to get him a job while Mom tended the store. Sometimes Dad was so tired after working a double shift that he would sleep in the back of his 1949 Willys Jeep wagon rather than risk driving, exhausted, all the way back home to Mountain City. I didn't see him a lot during that time. When Potter's Grocery became a money loser, they had to close it and look for another way to support us. (It seems that Mom and Dad had let their out-of-work customers, all of whom were neighbors and many of whom were relatives, run up tabs they could never pay off.)

After that, we lived in a duplex close to the glass plant until Mom and Dad had saved enough money to make a down payment on a rundown house a few miles outside of town that Dad would spend months fixing up.

Dad never knew much about his own father. One day when Dad was in the third grade, his father walked away and never came back, leaving my grandmother to raise nine children herself. They all had to get odd jobs to help put food on the table. When he was in his early twenties, Dad joined the Civilian Conservation Corps, a Great Depression–era work program created during the Roosevelt administration. The CCC put him on a train and sent him across the country to help build a public works project in Doty, Washington. He mailed almost everything he made back home to his mother, as he did later when the army sent him to Europe and North Africa during World War II.

Mom and Dad were introduced by Dad's older sister Frances and Mom's older brother Otho, who were married in the mid-1930s. Mom and Dad dated for years before the war but decided not go get married until Dad returned (they hoped) from his tour of duty. While Dad was overseas, Mom got a wartime job working on an assembly line at a chemical plant in Kingsport. They were married a few days after Dad got back home. I didn't arrive for another six years.

Neither of my parents was able to finish high school, having to work instead. They wanted nothing more than for me to have an easier life than they'd had, and they knew I wouldn't have a chance unless I had a good education. They sacrificed years to save enough money to send me to college. I will never be able to repay them or thank them enough.

I became the first person in my family to earn a college degree when I graduated from the University of Tennessee in 1973.

After a rocky start—I was far more interested in going to frat parties than attending lectures during my first few months in Knoxville—I finally settled into a good enough routine to begin making decent grades. I've had many lucky breaks over the years, but none luckier than being assigned an adviser named Sammie Lynn Puett. She had a reputation of being so strict that some of my fellow students in the College of Communications told me that if I were smart, I would get another adviser.

I did try, but the school wouldn't let me ditch Puett, for which I will always be grateful. She was indeed demanding, but she became my first-ever mentor. I soon realized that she was strict because she wanted her students to learn and to succeed. In addition to being my student adviser, she was my first journalism teacher. Believing that I might have some potential, she encouraged me to continue in journalism and to get a job at the student newspaper, the *Daily Beacon*. I did, and I fell in love with being a reporter. I spent more time in the *Daily Beacon* newsroom than anywhere else during my last two years at UT. I eventually worked myself up to editor during my senior year.

Puett always had a lot of irons in the fire, and one of her ambitions was to develop a first-class public relations program at the university. Like many other Puett groupies, I wanted to take every course she taught, even her PR courses. By the time I graduated, I had taken all the PR courses the university offered, including the graduate-level classes, and was torn between going into journalism and pursuing a public relations job when I left school. I was a charter member of the UT chapter of the Public Relations Society of America's student arm, and I helped drive a UT van carrying Puett and several other PR students to the 1972 PRSA national conference in Detroit.

Not once during that time did I get any training in how to set up a front group or mount a deception-based, fearmongering campaign for a client. I do remember discussions about the importance of behaving ethically in both journalism and PR—and the distinction between propaganda and "good" PR—but it never dawned on me then that I would ever do anything of which Puett would disapprove.

Journalism won over PR as my career choice because of Watergate. I fancied myself a great investigative reporter, maybe even the next Bob Woodward or Carl Bernstein. I had been lucky enough to get a summer internship between my junior and senior years at the *Memphis Press-Scimitar*, an afternoon paper. Offered a full-time job there after I got my B.A. in communications, I didn't think twice about accepting—even though by then I'd talked to a couple of PR agencies.

A few months into my career at the daily, I stumbled upon a great story about corruption in the city auto-inspection department. My reporting caught the attention of the managing editor, Ed Ray, and within months I was offered a job in the paper's Nashville bureau, covering the state legislature. Two years after that, I was promoted to Scripps Howard's Washington bureau. Scripps Howard owned the *Press-Scimitar* (which closed in 1983) as well as the *Commercial Appeal* in Memphis and the *News Sentinel* in Knoxville. So, at the age of twenty-four, I was covering Congress, the White House, and the Supreme Court.

AN INTRO TO PR LIKE NO OTHER

I liked Washington but, frankly, never got over being homesick for Tennessee. In 1978, a college friend introduced me to a wealthy Knoxville banker by the name of Jake Butcher, who was running for governor of Tennessee. When Butcher asked me to be his press secretary, I took the job, seeing it as a ticket back home. Butcher won the Democratic primary but lost the general election to Lamar Alexander, now the senior senator from Tennessee. (I was devastated when Butcher lost, but it was probably a good thing for the state that he did, because five years later his banking empire collapsed and he went to jail on bank fraud charges.)

I continued to work for Butcher after the campaign—in a very different role. As it turned out, Butcher (whose brother, C. H., also had a growing banking empire, which stretched from Kentucky to Georgia) headed a group of civic and business leaders trying to bring a World's Fair to Knoxville. He asked me if I would be interested in working in one of his banks and doing some lobbying and PR work for the World's Fair group. Not having anything else lined up after the campaign, I agreed.

It was a great gig while it lasted. I represented the group in Washington as a lobbyist because the Bureau of International Expositions, in Paris (which decides where World's Fairs are held), insists that a city have its federal government's backing and financial support before even being considered. After helping secure a congressional authorization for the fair, I got to travel around the world helping recruit countries to participate in it. The event itself, the 1982 World's Fair and Energy Exhibition, was a six-month blast. I wrote speeches and press releases for Butcher, but mostly just had a great time hanging out with the Australians and Peruvians and Egyptians. My wife, a Knoxville native whom I met in Washington while I was lobbying, even got a job as manager of the Egyptian pavilion.

After the fair closed in October 1982, I continued to work in the PR department of Jake Butcher's flagship bank in Knoxville, United American. Everything fell apart four months later—and ten days after our first child was born. Federal and state bank examiners were suspicious that the Butchers were moving problem loans from one bank to another to avoid detection. The Feds decided to mount a massive examination of all the Butcher banks at once, and they found what they were looking for. After attempts by Governor Alexander and others to keep the banks from failing, regulators shut them down on Valentine's Day in 1983. One of C. H. Butcher's banks was a savings bank not insured by the FDIC, meaning that thousands of people lost their life savings. Hundreds of people, including me, lost their jobs. It was a heck of a learning experience. As the spokesman for a failing banking empire, I learned the hard way what crisis communications was all about.

Luck smiled on me again, though, a few months after that. The Butchers had hired Hill & Knowlton Public Relations to help with both the fair and the bank, and I had gotten to know a lot of the firm's executives in Chicago and Atlanta. Two of the Atlanta account executives, Kay McKenzie and Betty Rider Gordon, decided to hang out their own shingle, and they invited me to join them. Once again, having nothing else lined up, I said yes, and I moved to Atlanta with my family and helped launch McKenzie, Gordon, and Potter.

We made a good go of it for a few years, but eventually we dissolved the partnership. My family and I moved back to Knoxville, and I took a job as head of PR and advertising for the nonprofit and church-affiliated Baptist Health System of East Tennessee, which comprised three hospitals, a few clinics, and an HMO. I don't think I'd ever heard of an HMO until then, but all of a sudden I was the PR guy for one. After doing that for a couple of years, I was given a chance to make a lot more money by moving to Louisville, Kentucky, and joining the PR team at Humana, a big for-profit company. At that time, in 1989, Humana had a huge division that owned and operated scores of hospitals in the United States and Europe and another division that operated managed care plans.

One of the executives at Baptist begged me not to go "to the dark side," meaning cross over to for-profit health care. But I didn't fully understand yet how different it would be, and I saw it as a great career opportunity. Taking a well-paying job with great benefits at a *Fortune* 500 company seemed like a no-brainer.

So, it was off to Louisville (four of us this time: myself, my wife, our six-year-old son, and our two-year-old daughter) for my first exposure to the corporate world. I adapted well and was pretty proud to be working for one of the city's biggest and most prominent employers in the city's most conspicuous office building: a twenty-seven-story Michael Graves–designed postmodern pink-granite skyscraper with a pair of Giacometti sculptures in the lobby. My digs at Baptist were nothing compared to my office in the Humana building.

I supported the hospital division until Humana decided that operating both hospitals and managed care plans wasn't working out as planned. For the hospitals to make money, they had to have a steady stream of paying patients. For the managed care plans to make money, they had to keep people out of the hospital—including Humana's hospitals. When investors and Wall Street analysts told Humana's executives that they needed to focus on one business and sell the other, they decided to spin off the hospitals. I was asked to stay with Humana, now a managed care company, and soon became head of communications.

MY TRIP TO THE MAJOR LEAGUES

A few months later, I got a call from another recruiter about an even better, higher-paying, and more prestigious job in Connecticut. How could I say no to CIGNA, one of the biggest and most highly respected insurers in the country?

CIGNA in 1993, the year I joined the company, was a large multi-line insurer that traced its roots back to the eighteenth century, when a predecessor company, Insurance Company of North America (INA), started selling fire and marine insurance in Philadelphia. This historic company merged in 1982 with the Connecticut General Insurance Company, known as Connecticut General (CG). (The name CIGNA is an anagram of the acronyms of the two companies.)

Although it was much larger than Humana and had become a big player in managed care as a result of acquisitions, CIGNA was still known primarily as a property and casualty company. I was hired to help boost awareness of CIGNA's health care business. Moving from Kentucky to Connecticut (where CIGNA's health care operations are based) and from Humana to CIGNA really felt like moving to the major leagues.

I hit a home run about a year after signing on when I arranged for a reporter with *Modern Healthcare*, the leading industry trade magazine, to do a big feature story on CIGNA. She wanted to "look under the hood" of a managed care company but hadn't been able to get any of the others to let her do it. After persuading senior management that it would be worth the risk, I invited her to Bloomfield, Connecticut, to spend a day with us. I, of course, had spent many hours preparing the executives she would interview and made sure she only talked to people on an approved list. She was so appreciative that she wrote a glowing multipage story about the company and its "customer-focused" approach to managed care. It was so popular among CIGNA's sales force that I couldn't keep enough reprints in stock. Within three months, they ordered thirty thousand copies of the story to send to clients and use in sales presentations.

I also got noticed for developing a "rapid response" approach to handling media calls about member complaints, which we called "horror stories." I worked closely with the chief medical officer to set up a kind of SWAT team to be called into action at a moment's notice when a reporter called with a potential horror story. The objective was to get as much information as possible—as soon as possible—about the complaining member so my team and I could respond to the reporter with a statement or background information before the reporter's deadline. We were able to keep many stories out of print or off the air just by being so unusually attentive to reporters when they called. It was media relations at its best, at least for CIGNA.

One of the horror stories that we could not keep from being published, and that led to the creation of our rapid-response system, appeared in the *Hartford Courant* on August 8, 1996, under the headline

"New Health Care Concern: Drive-Through Mastectomies." Reporter Diane Levick, one of the country's most knowledgeable and aggressive health care journalists, reported that at least two HMOs in Connecticut were requiring hospitals to discharge breast cancer patients on the same day they underwent a mastectomy unless their surgeon could prove that an overnight stay was "medically necessary." The two HMOs were CIGNA and ConnectiCare.

The HMOs had instituted the discharge guidelines after an actuarial firm that publishes guidelines on medical practices and procedures had noted that mastectomies were being done in some parts of the country on an outpatient basis. The move outraged local surgeons and lawmakers. After Levick broke the story, dozens of other reporters did similar stories across the country.

Word of these "drive-through mastectomies" and of "drive-through deliveries" (insurers were also telling hospitals to discharge new mothers on the same day they had their baby) touched off a national backlash against HMOs that led to laws in many states mandating a stay of at least one overnight for breast-surgery patients and new mothers.

In 1997, after handling dozens of horror stories and keeping many others out of the media, I was rewarded with a promotion to the corporate PR staff, which meant I would have to relocate my family from Connecticut to Philadelphia. They were not happy to leave our home in West Hartford, but the increase in salary was too good to turn down. I thrived in my new role, and by 2002 I was leading the corporate communications department. When I left the company in May 2008, I was its top PR executive.

During my years at CIGNA, in addition to my responsibilities at the company, I became increasingly active at the industry level. I really felt I had arrived at the top of my profession when I became a regular on the Amtrak Metroliner to Washington. I worked closely with my counterparts at other big insurers on numerous trade association committees and task forces. We often met at the offices of the PR firms we hired to set up coalitions and front groups to promote the industry's political agenda, which was mostly an ongoing effort to keep what the industry considered "anti-managed-care legislation" from being enacted.

By then, the HMO backlash had reached Congress, and several bills were introduced every year to force insurers to change or stop using entirely many of the practices that enabled them to pay less for medical care, such as refusing to include certain doctors and hospitals in their provider networks and refusing to pay for certain doctor-ordered care unless they could be convinced that it was necessary. To ensure that the bills would never pass, my peers and I hired some of Washington's biggest PR firms to plan and implement stealth campaigns to manipulate public opinion on one issue or another as part of a broader strategy to kill any legislation the industry didn't like.

One of the most successful stealth campaigns we launched was in response to bipartisan efforts in Congress to pass a Patient's Bill of Rights. The insurance industry was opposed to many of the consumer protections in the bill, one of which would have forced insurers to make an external review process available to enrollees who were denied coverage for doctor-ordered treatments. Insurers also didn't like the fact that the bill would have given enrollees an expanded right to sue their insurer and employer for wrongful denials of coverage. Using a PR firm, Porter Novelli, we formed a front group called the Health Benefits Coalition, which conducted a fearmongering campaign to convince the public—and lawmakers—that enactment of a Patient's Bill of Rights would lead to a tidal wave of frivolous lawsuits that would cause health insurance premiums to skyrocket.

I didn't feel then that we were doing anything unethical or underhanded. We were all well read and well educated and could hold our own at any cocktail party, regardless of the subject. We were charming and articulate and sophisticated. We all wore nice clothes and ate at the best restaurants and had kids in good schools and houses in the right zip codes. We knew people in Congress and the White House.

We talked every day to reporters at the *Wall Street Journal* and the *New York Times*. We were powerful and influential—not nearly as much so as our CEOs, of course, but what we did and said mattered. The American dream didn't get any better than this.

In my job, I talked about people who were uninsured, but only in terms of their numbers. They were all numbers—they didn't have names or faces or families. I also talked about CIGNA's millions of members—who likewise had no names or faces or families.

I talked about the billions of dollars in premiums and fees that CIGNA took in from those millions of members and the hundreds of millions of dollars that the company earned from these premiums and fees every single quarter.

I talked about the company's business model and things like earnings per share and the medical-loss ratio and what was going on in Washington.

I lived and worked in this abstract world, far away from my days on Spear Branch Road and in Kingsport. But I had begun to ask myself whether managed care—especially as it was being administered by big for-profit corporations—was really the solution to the country's worsening health crisis.

It took a movie, a trip back home to Tennessee, and the tragic death of a seventeen-year-old girl—just three years younger than my own daughter—for me to see that it was not.

What happened next made me see the world and the work I was doing from an entirely different perspective. I was about to undergo a fundamental shift that would change the direction of my life.

CHAPTER II

The Campaign Against *Sicko*

MOST of the two thousand people who crowded into the Grand Théâtre Lumière at the Cannes Film Festival early on Saturday morning, May 19, 2007, for the world premiere of *Sicko*, Michael Moore's indictment of the U.S. health care system, rose to their feet at the end of the film and gave Moore and his new documentary an astonishing fifteen-minute standing ovation.

One young man, however, could not stay to applaud because of an urgent assignment. Largely unnoticed, he slipped out of the theater and made his way to his hotel room, where he placed a call to the organization in Washington, D.C., that not only had covered his trip to the French Riviera and his ticket to the premiere but also paid his salary.

Dialing America's Health Insurance Plans, he was immediately patched into a conference call where dozens of insurance executives, including me, waited anxiously on the line. All knew of the threat to the industry; none knew any specifics. Moore had kept such tight control over the release of his film that none of us knew exactly what it was about. Would it focus on big pharmaceutical companies, as early rumors had suggested, or on the insurance industry?

As he read from the extensive notes he had taken in the back of the dark theater, AHIP's reconnaissance agent confirmed our worst fears: Private health insurance companies played the role of the villain.

Which companies were in the movie, we wanted to know, and how badly were they portrayed?

I was cautiously optimistic. Because there had not been a single Moore sighting at any of CIGNA's facilities or any reports that he had interviewed anyone associated with the company, I thought there was a good chance he had chosen other targets. I was hoping especially that archrival Aetna had been in his sights.

But I was wrong: CIGNA was among the first companies in the line of fire. My phone would soon be ringing off the hook with calls from reporters and TV producers wanting to get my reaction to the claims of people in the film who said we had refused to pay for needed medical care. I also knew, though, that I would get a lot of support from AHIP, which was poised to mount a massive PR campaign to discredit Moore and his movie.

Industry leaders had already agreed to provide the resources for a campaign to attack the movie because of the concern that it would persuade more Americans to support a Medicare-for-all, government-run health care system that would marginalize, if not eliminate, the role of private insurance companies. Industry-commissioned polls had been showing for several years that many Americans, worried about rapidly rising insurance premiums and reports of insurance companies refusing to pay for necessary medical treatments, were not as opposed to such a system as they used to be. Several years had passed since the fear-based propaganda campaigns financed by special interests had scared Americans away from Bill and Hillary Clinton's health care reform proposal. There had been only occasional need for fear-mongering during the industry-friendly Bush years.

Another big concern was the timing of Moore's film. The campaigns for the Democratic and Republican presidential nominations were in full swing. If Moore's movie attracted big audiences and generated a lot of positive buzz, it might embolden one or more

Democratic candidates to join Representative Dennis Kucinich (D-Ohio) in endorsing the expansion of Medicare to cover everybody. If the man or woman elected in 2008 favored such a radical restructuring of the American health care system, the increasingly profitable insurance industry would find itself in a war for survival.

After hearing the report from Cannes, we knew that was a real possibility. Moore's movie compared the U.S. system, dominated by large for-profit insurance companies, with the nonprofit, government-run systems of Canada, France, the United Kingdom, and even Cuba, all of which have attained universal coverage for their citizens while spending far less for care that's as good as, if not better than, the care Americans receive. Not surprisingly, considering the anticorporate theme of Moore's previous documentaries, the U.S. system did not fare well in the comparison.

AHIP—and every PR person in the health insurance industry—had been trying to get information about Moore's intentions since July 2004, when he had mentioned to a reporter that his next film would be about the U.S. health care system. Most of us had feared it was just a matter of time before he and his film crew began showing up at our corporate headquarters demanding to talk to our CEOs, or worse, waiting at their homes.

In anticipation of those tactics—which he had used in most of his other films—I met with corporate security to develop a plan to make sure that managers at every CIGNA office knew what to do in the event that Moore showed up at their doorstep. I also scheduled media-training sessions with all of the company's top executives, equipping them with pithy things to say and pointers on how not to look like a deer caught in the headlights if they got ambushed leaving their home or getting out of their limo.

Above all, we in the industry strove to keep our activities and plans close to the vest. Fearful that an internal memo or e-mail might be leaked to the media or wind up in Moore's hands, AHIP advised all of its member companies not to put Moore's name or anything remotely related to his project in writing. AHIP didn't want insurance companies to appear to be on the defensive. In December 2004, it was disclosed that at least six drug companies had been warning their employees, in internal e-mails, to keep an eye out for Moore. When one of the e-mails was leaked, Moore went straight to the media with it, knowing that the drug companies had unwittingly given him exactly what he needed to generate early interest in his movie.

Determined to avoid the same scenario, insurers were giving their employees the same instructions, but not in writing. AHIP was so cautious that its staff was instructed to use the code term "Hollywood" in communications to company executives about Moore and his movie.

In one of her few written communications about Moore, AHIP president Karen Ignagni sent a note to her board of directors in late 2004 about "health care and Hollywood." Ignagni had charged AHIP's communications staff and PR agencies with the task of searching for every mention of the movie they could find, and they had come across a brief story in the blog Cinematical, which read in part, "Though he's clearly passionate about exposing the problems with American health care, Moore still seems to be struggling a bit with the film—after all, he says, 'everyone knows that health care is a mess in this country.' His goal, then, seems to be less education than motivation: Moore hopes that [Sicko] 'pushes health care to the top of the public agenda' and, presumably, forces politicians to get involved."

IT NEVER HURTS TO PLAN AHEAD

In late May 2007, ten days after Sicko's Cannes premiere, the top public relations executives of the country's biggest health insurers flew to Philadelphia to be briefed on AHIP's multipronged strategy to discredit both Moore and his movie.

The meeting was being held in Philadelphia instead of Washington because the chair of AHIP's Strategic Communications

Committee was CIGNA's CEO, H. Edward Hanway, and he wanted to host the meeting close to home. It was the second time in two weeks that the group had met there. Three days before *Sicko's* premiere, they had convened to hear Bill McInturff, partner and cofounder of Public Opinion Strategies, a national Republican and corporate research firm, disclose the results of four focus groups and three national polls his firm had conducted for AHIP in recent months to determine Americans' attitudes on the need for health care reform.

McInturff, who was later to be lead pollster for the 2008 McCain-Palin campaign, has had a long association with the health insurance industry, going back to the early 1990s. He earned his chops when he teamed up with the political consultants and creative team at ad agency Goddard Claussen to create the "Harry and Louise" commercials, which helped scuttle the Clinton health care reform plan in 1994. He has played a key role ever since in helping the industry defeat any federal legislation that has posed a serious threat to insurers' profitability.

Much of McInturff's work has been devoted to what he describes as "'combat message development,' not simply monitoring public opinion, but developing messages to defend and promote client interests on complex public policy issues."

McInturff began his presentation by making it clear—and showing the evidence—that Americans were rapidly losing confidence in the private health insurance market. His first slide showed that there had been a significant shift in recent years and that a majority of people, according to his polls, were now saying the government should do more to solve the many problems that plagued the American health care system. Even more troublesome, a fast-growing percentage also embraced the idea that a government-run, publicly funded health care system—like the ones Moore portrayed in *Sicko*—should be implemented in the United States.

As a result of this trend and in anticipation of the first national debate on reforming the health care system since insurers had played a key role in killing the Clinton reform plan, AHIP had recently restructured its Strategic Communications Committee to include only CEOs. It had originally been made up of member companies' top PR people, and I had served on the committee as CIGNA's representative, but AHIP's board reasoned that the committee's recommendations would have greater clout throughout the industry if CEOs were perceived to have created them. (The PR chiefs, including me and my peers from the other companies that would be attending the second Philadelphia meeting, now comprised the Strategic Communications *Advisory* Committee.)

Also traveling to Philadelphia for the meeting were AHIP's Mike Tuffin and Robert Schooling, senior vice president of the Washington-based PR firm APCO Worldwide. Tuffin and Schooling would be the main presenters of the industry's strategy against *Sicko*.

APCO was founded in 1984 by one of Washington's biggest law firms, Arnold & Porter, which is well known for its representation of the tobacco industry. From one office in Washington, APCO has grown into an international operation with offices in twenty-nine locations throughout North America, Europe, Asia, and Africa. On its Web site, APCO has referred to itself as "a global communications consultancy" specializing in "influencing decision-makers and shaping public opinion by crafting compelling messages and recruiting effective allies."

One of the deceptive practices of which APCO has a long history is setting up and running front groups for its clients. In 1993, Philip Morris hired APCO to organize a front group called the Advancement of Sound Science Coalition in response to the U.S. Environmental Protection Agency's ruling that secondhand tobacco smoke was a carcinogen. Philip Morris also hired APCO to manage what it called a "massive national effort aimed at altering the American judicial system to be more hostile toward product liability suits" and to build a coalition to advocate for tort reform. According to the Center for Media and Democracy, the tobacco industry paid APCO almost a million dollars in 1995 to implement behind-the-scenes tort reform efforts and specifically to create chapters of "grassroots" citizens' groups called Citizens Against Lawsuit Abuse.

A 1995 APCO pamphlet described how the firm helped corporations advance their goals by influencing lawmakers, drafting legislation and regulations, and creating business coalitions tailored to specific issues: "We [APCO] use the most effective, up-to-date technology and campaign tactics to help you achieve your legislative and regulatory goals . . . [We have] built numerous national and state coalitions on a variety of issues including the environment, science, energy, trade, intellectual property, education, tort reform and health care . . . [We] apply tactics usually reserved for political campaigns to target audiences and recruit third-party advocates. Our staff has the political field experience and has written the direct mail, managed the telephones, crafted the television commercials and trained the grassroots volunteers. We apply these hard-learned skills and tactics to mobilize hundreds, even thousands, of constituents. Or, when just the 'grasstops' are needed, we recruit just a few of a target's key friends or contributors to join us. No matter the issue, we bring together coalitions that are credible, persuasive and cost-effective."

While APCO mentions some of its clients on its Web site under the heading of "Client Success," it doesn't disclose all of them. You will find no mention of AHIP there. That's because AHIP does not want the public to know anything about the PR strategies the firm creates and the front groups it sets up for the insurance industry.

At the time of the Philadelphia meeting, Tuffin had recently returned to AHIP from APCO, where he had served as a top account executive whose clients had included the pharmaceutical industry. Before APCO and his first stint at AHIP, he'd been the senior director of strategic communications at the trade group Pharmaceutical Researchers and Manufacturers of America and, earlier, the communications director at GOPAC, a Republican political action committee.

Schooling, who had joined APCO in 1995 after working as a senior field director for the National Association of Homebuilders, came from the other side of the political aisle. In the early part of his career, he had been a field director for the Democratic Congressional Campaign Committee.

For the strategy meeting, AHIP had encouraged the PR people to attend in person rather than calling in. It did not want to risk the chance that anyone other than those specifically invited would be able to hear how the industry planned to discredit Moore and his film. Secrecy was paramount. There would be no handouts. A secure conference call line was set up for those few who could not attend in person, and they were given passwords—but only after the meeting started—so they could view the PowerPoint presentations on their office computers. The "save" and "print" functions were disabled so that no one could keep any evidence, other than their own handwritten notes, that the meeting had taken place.

To drive the point home, the first slide of the presentation warned that any communications we disseminated in writing, even to employees, could wind up on Moore's Web site.

Though the movie would not reach American screens for another month, AHIP and APCO had created a comprehensive PR campaign, elements of which, we were to learn, were already being implemented.

The initial thrust of the campaign would be an attempt to shift the media's focus away from Moore's agenda as much as possible and to position health insurers as part of the solution rather than part of the problem. Tuffin said that when any of us talked to the media about *Sicko*, we should acknowledge the compelling stories and personal tragedies in the film but then try to change the subject to how insurers contribute to the American health care system.

Schooling added that it was imperative for all of us to redouble our efforts to educate the public on the positive things the industry does. Hanway suggested that every company should begin collecting positive stories to counter the negative ones in the movie. Schooling said that APCO would work with any company's PR team to help place positive stories in the media. While this effort was under way, APCO would work behind the scenes to "reframe the debate" by mounting a campaign against government-run health care systems. Schooling said the strategy to do that would be bifurcated. On the one hand, insurers would need to stay on message by continuing to talk about how they can help solve problems relating to access, cost, and quality of care. On the other hand, AHIP and APCO would recruit allies to communicate what industry spokespeople could not do with credibility—that Moore was a nut whose ideas on reform would be a disaster for the country.

Tuffin and Schooling said they had already begun recruiting conservative and free-market think tanks, including the American Enterprise Institute and the Galen Institute, as third-party allies. Those allies, they said, would be working aggressively to discredit Moore and his movie.

They then mentioned an ally that most of us had never heard of, Health Care America. It had been created by AHIP and APCO for the sole purpose of attacking Moore and his contention that people in countries with government-run systems spent far less and got better care than people in the United States. The sole reason Health Care America exists, they said, was to talk about the shortcomings of government-run systems.

Unlike the Galen Institute and AEI, Health Care America was a front group, funded by money from the health insurance industry and other special interests, that APCO would set up and run out of its offices. Although Schooling didn't disclose this at the meeting, the person who would serve as the media contact for Health Care America would be APCO employee Bill Pierce, a man who had served in the top communications job at the Blue Cross and Blue Shield Association, another insurance trade group, and as a public affairs officer at the Department of Health and Human Services during the George W. Bush administration, before joining APCO as a senior vice president.

Creating Health Care America—which would spring into action as soon as *Sicko* hit theaters in the United States—was deemed necessary because of the steady and alarming erosion in Amerians' opposition to government-run systems, as borne out by McInturff's research. Health Care America would lead the effort to restore Americans' fear of government-run health care.

While Health Care America and the industry's allies would be doing the fearmongering, AHIP and insurers would try to persuade the public as well as lawmakers that the industry had a legitimate reason to exist. One of the key messages AHIP would stress in every media interview about health care reform during the coming months was that this time the industry would be "bringing solutions to the table," and would be willing to make certain concessions when Congress began drafting reform legislation. This would be the part of its PR charm offensive that insurers would want the public to see.

The part they would not want the public to see, however, was their effort to depict Moore as such a polarizing figure—loved by left-wingers and liberal activists but viewed with suspicion by more conservative voters—that Democrats would talk positively about *Sicko* at their own peril. The goal was to make Moore radioactive to centrist Democrats in particular. The plan included recruiting political pundits, including some Democrats, to articulate that threat. AHIP and APCO would also reach out to political reporters and try to frame the movie as an effort on the part of Moore and other liberals to drive the agenda to the political left.

Tuffin and Schooling wrapped up their presentation with a "worst-case scenario" plan. If *Sicko* showed signs of being as influential in shaping public opinion on health care reform as *An Inconvenient Truth* had been in changing attitudes about climate change, then the industry would have to consider implementing a plan "to push Moore off the cliff." They didn't elaborate, and no one asked what they meant by that. We knew they didn't mean it literally—that a hit man would be sent to take Moore out. Rather, an all-out effort would be made to depict

Moore as someone intent on destroying the free-market health care system and with it, the American way of life.

TOO BAD THE CIA ISN'T THIS EFFICIENT

A few days later, my assistant brought me a one-and-a-half-inch-thick unmarked three-ring binder. The only indications that it came from AHIP were a few references in the table of contents to a white paper the organization had produced on the Canadian health care system and a few other documents on AHIP's reform proposals.

The binder contained responses to just about any conceivable question a reporter might ask about the movie or government-run systems, but in keeping with AHIP's ban on even mentioning Moore or *Sicko* in writing, there were no specific references to either. AHIP sent the binder to all of the PR chiefs who participated in the Philadelphia meeting to equip us with negative anecdotes and statistics about any of the health care systems depicted in *Sicko* and to remind us to always mention in our conversations with anyone about the movie that Americans do not want a government takeover of their health care system.

The phrase "government takeover" is one that has tested extremely well over the years and has been central to every campaign the industry has conducted in recent decades to defeat reform efforts, including the Clinton proposal in 1994. The industry has paid McInturff and other consultants and pollsters millions of dollars to craft and test such phrases in focus groups and surveys. Knowing from that research that many Americans react negatively to more government involvement in their lives, particularly if it involves higher taxes, AHIP ensured that a warning against a government takeover was included in the briefing packets for lawmakers in Washington, the industry's business allies, and conservative pundits, talk show hosts, and editorial writers.

Two weeks after the Philadelphia meeting, I was on a cross-country reconnaissance mission of my own. Although the AHIP staffer who saw the movie in Cannes provided a pretty good report, he did not give many details about how CIGNA was portrayed in the film.

After hearing that the first public screening of the movie would be held in Sacramento on June 12, I asked the head of our state government affairs unit if she could finagle a ticket for me. I wanted to be as prepared as possible to answer questions from the media when they began to flood in. The best way to do that would be to see the movie myself. Terry McGann, CIGNA's longtime lobbyist in Sacramento, was able to score a couple of tickets for a colleague and me from California State Assembly speaker Fabian Núñez, a Democrat from Los Angeles.

The screening was an unofficial premiere. The official premiere would be held four days later in the Michigan town of Bellaire, which is near where Moore and his wife live. Moore had been persuaded by the California Nurses Association and Physicians for a National Health Program—both advocates of a single-payer health care system in the United States—to show the movie in Sacramento first because California lawmakers had twice approved bills creating a single-payer system in the state. Had Governor Arnold Schwarzenegger not vetoed both bills, California would have been the first state in the nation to ban private insurance companies and operate its own government-run health care system, like many of those depicted in *Sicko*.

After picking up our tickets in McGann's office, my colleague and I walked to the theater, trying to blend in with the thousands of politicians, state government employees, doctors, and nurses who were already in line to see the movie. Once inside, we went to the very back row and took out our pens and notebooks, ready to capture the details of the stories told in the movie by people who claimed that CIGNA had refused to pay for care their doctors had said they needed.

It seemed as if there were more stories about CIGNA than about any other company, although I didn't pay as much attention to how badly Moore treated our competitors. Probably one of the most memorable vignettes in the whole movie was about a hearing-impaired little girl, Annette Noe, whose doctors said she needed cochlear implants in both of her ears. CIGNA initially paid for only one, saying that implantation in both ears would be "too experimental." The girl's father, Doug Noe, was one of twenty-five thousand people who had responded to Moore's call for health insurance horror stories. Undoubtedly, one of the reasons Annette's story made it into the movie is that her father told the CIGNA representative he had been dealing with that he had been in touch with Moore.

"Has your CEO ever been in a movie?" Noe asked the CIGNA guy.

The next scene showed CIGNA's fifty-eight-story glass-sheathed headquarters in Philadelphia, where I worked. What viewers heard next was the CIGNA representative calling back and leaving good news on the Noes' answering machine. CIGNA would pay for both implants after all.

I cringed when I heard that, but I wasn't surprised. The squeaky wheel gets the grease in the managed care world. That wasn't the first time CIGNA had delivered good news after a member had complained to the media about a denial. It would not be the last, either.

But the movie had an effect on me that I didn't expect. Because of all the experience I'd had handling "horror stories" like the ones depicted, I knew that they were a common occurrence—that many Americans found themselves in similar situations every day. I also found the film very moving and very effective in its condemnation of the practices of private health insurance companies. There were many times when I had to fight to hold back tears. Moore had gotten it right. If I hadn't been with a colleague, I probably would have joined all the others in the audience in giving the movie a standing ovation, just as the people at Cannes did when it was first screened.

The next day, the front group that APCO had set up to discredit *Sicko* issued a statement warning against "a government takeover" of health care:

"Health Care America, a non-partisan, non-profit health care advocacy organization, released the following statement in response to a California rally held by Michael Moore and a variety of advocates in support of a government takeover of our health care system.

"The reality is that government-run health systems around the world are failing patients—forcing them to forgo treatments or seek out-of-pocket care in other countries."

Bill Pierce was listed as the contact person for Health Care America, but if you had dialed the phone number listed for him at the organization, you would have reached him at his desk at APCO in Washington.

A week later, Moore held another screening, this one in Washington. He invited members of Congress, but few showed up. He also invited the heads of the big health care trade associations. None of them attended.

The industry, however, was prepared for the event. An ad targeting the movie appeared in Washington's newspapers. The message: "In America, you wait in line to see a movie. In government-run health care systems, you wait to see a doctor." The sponsor: Health Care America.

For several weeks after that screening, APCO sent me and other PR chiefs daily reports of the stories it had placed in the media via Health Care America as well as the commentaries and op-eds APCO's recruits had had published in newspapers and other media outlets from coast to coast.

The campaign cost hundreds of thousands of dollars, all of which came from premiums paid by health-plan members, but industry executives felt this was a good and appropriate use of those premium dollars. Though *Sicko* grossed nearly $25 million at the box office in the United States, that figure wasn't even in the same ballpark as the $120 million that Moore's *Fahrenheit 9/11* had made on U.S. screens just three years earlier. We believed the industry's behind-the-scenes campaign against the movie might have had something to do with the comparatively small box office numbers. We were pleased that AHIP and

APCO had succeeded in getting their talking points into most of the stories that appeared about the movie, and that not a single reporter had done enough investigative work to find out that insurers had provided the lion's share of funding to set up Health Care America.

We were also relieved that centrist Democrats had not embraced *Sicko*. All in all, the movie, in our view, had not succeeded in altering the "collective opinion." Spending the extra money to push Moore off the cliff had not been necessary.

More important, we considered the campaign against *Sicko* to be a warm-up act to the health care reform debate that all of us knew would begin in Congress soon after the next president took office. And most of us still believed that person would be the industry's former nemesis, Hillary Clinton.

CHAPTER III

Perception Is Reality

BEFORE I take you with me on my unexpectedly life-changing trip to Tennessee and describe the last horror story I ever worked on for CIGNA, I should explain how public relations evolved into such a powerful yet largely invisible force in our society. I also want to give you an idea of what I actually did on a day-to-day basis as head of PR at one of the country's biggest insurers.

To understand why you believe some of the things you believe and do some of the things you do, it's important for you to understand what PR people do and how they do it.

It's actually nothing new. Human beings have distorted information for as long as they've communicated—with gestures, sounds, nuanced words, or whatever it takes to bring other people around. Whether it's as brazen as a pyramid or as subtle as a white lie, this art form—often called spin—has become as much a part of our culture as the media we depend upon to connect and inform us.

The "spin doctors" who shape much of what we see and read today are often shadowy figures in the multi-billion-dollar industry we call "public relations." The most successful of them hobnob with royalty and presidents, CEOs and movie stars. They are experts in every medium, and they use their considerable resources to build and maintain strong, positive images for their clients. They cultivate contacts and relationships among journalists and other media gatekeepers. They walk a fine line between contributing to the so-called marketplace of ideas and warping public understanding to their clients' ends. Oftentimes, this line is so creatively blurred as to disappear.

What exactly is PR? What are the boundaries, the restrictions, the rules? The first question is easier to answer. *Cutlip & Center's Effective Public Relations*, the encyclopedia, if not the bible, of the industry, defines PR as "the management function that establishes and maintains mutually beneficial relationships between an organization and the publics on whom its success or failure depends."[1] That definition emphasizes the two-way nature of PR, as opposed to the one-way communication that characterizes propaganda or advertising.

The Public Relations Society of America describes what PR does rather than what it is: "Public relations helps an organization and its publics adapt mutually to each other."[2] Again, an emphasis on two-way exchange, although PRSA's highest organizational award is the Silver Anvil, "symbolizing the forging of public opinion." Either way, PR is the middleman, whose loyalty to the client often supersedes everything else.

To be sure, PR has been—and is being—used to good ends. Even the noblest of causes can benefit from the services of a communications expert to clarify facts, disseminate information, and counter unfair arguments. And there are plenty of ethical PR people out there to do this.

But with PR so intricately woven into every major industry and movement in today's mass media reality, the stakes of spin have become incredibly high. And ethics do slip. PR often crosses the line into misleading, withholding, or simply lying. And when it does, society suffers—sometimes tragically so.

THE BEGINNING OF SPINNING

In what may be the first recorded discourse on public relations, Aristotle spoke of "rhetoric" in ancient Athens and urged that everyone be taught how to use it in order to tell truth from lies. His insight remained relevant over the millennia as the methods for distorting information evolved everywhere in the world. For example, in eighteenth-century Russia, Grigory Potemkin went to extremes on behalf of his empress (and supposed lover), Catherine the Great. A field marshal and adviser to Catherine, Potemkin made sure foreign leaders were impressed when they visited Russia by having artificial villages built throughout the countryside to create the impression of growth and prosperity. In so doing, he unwittingly ensured that his name would live throughout the ages—the term "Potemkin village" is still used to describe things that falsely imply substance.

Gossip, innuendo, and deception were common in publications and politics in the earliest years of the United States. Businesses manipulated the new nation's mass media as early as the 1830s, when the *New York Sun*, one of the early penny presses, offered to publish free "puff" stories (promotional material presented as regular news) for its advertisers. In the same period, American showman P. T. Barnum regularly pushed the limits of spin to a point that seems shocking even today. Barnum had no qualms about inventing outrageous claims and carrying them as far as possible by way of promoting his business or himself. In 1836, he "bought" an elderly woman—a slave named Joice Heth—and claimed she was the 161-year-old nursemaid to George Washington. When she died and doctors estimated her age to be only 80, Barnum said he was "shocked, deeply shocked" at the deception visited upon him.[3]

While Barnum was exceptional as his own promoter, it was publicists and press agents who handled most of the functions that would come to be grouped under the banner of PR, which emerged as a defined, distinctly American profession in the early twentieth century.

As I noted earlier, one of the first and most notable public relations men was Ivy Lee, who is credited with developing the concept of "crisis management," the organized, orchestrated communications response to a negative event—one of the basic practices of today's

PR. Lee, born in 1877 to a Methodist minister, graduated from Princeton and worked as a reporter for several newspapers, including the *New York Times*, before cofounding the Parker & Lee agency in New York.

While working for a group of coal mine operators in 1906, Lee seized an opportunity to define his agency's role and increase his credibility. Going against the prevalent Wall Street attitude that "the public be damned," Lee issued his famous "Declaration of Principles," emphasizing the public's need for accurate information. The statement (now part and parcel of most modern public relations textbooks) proved to be a milestone in establishing the new field of PR—separating it from the old image of publicity pushers, who by then were considered little more than hucksters and snake oil salesmen.[4] The declaration, which Lee sent to newspapers, read in part, "This is not a secret press bureau. All our work is done in the open. We aim to supply news . . . In brief, our plan is, frankly, and openly, on behalf of business concerns and public institutions, to supply to the press and public of the United States prompt and accurate information concerning subjects which it is of value and interest to the public to know about."

Lee's approach made it "easy" for reporters to cover a coal miners' strike against his clients. Rather than dodge their questions, Lee issued handouts, which came to be known as press releases, during each strike—and reporters responded by using them to create positive coverage about the mining companies. As his reputation grew, Lee attracted new clients, including John D. Rockefeller Sr., who hired him as an adviser in 1914.

Rockefeller was being vilified for the strike-breaking tactics of his Colorado Fuel and Iron Company against miners in Colorado. People were using terms like "Ludlow Massacre" and "Bloody Ludlow" to describe a company-sponsored offensive against strikers that killed not only miners but also women and children. Lee's first assignment was to diffuse public outrage. Among other things, he reduced public opposition by producing pro-company bulletins with titles like "The Struggle in Colorado for Industrial Freedom." Concurrently, Lee reportedly advised Rockefeller to improve his personal image by carrying dimes in his pockets and giving them to children in public.

Lee worked for Rockefeller again years later, this time in the wake of full-blown battles against striking coal miners in West Virginia. After seventy miners were killed, Lee turned once more to publishing bulletins that portrayed his client in a positive light. They emphasized the charitable work of mine owners and claimed that company stores—the only places where miners were able to spend the scrip they received as wages—were in business not to force miners to return their earnings to the company, but to help protect the hapless miners' assets.

The approach worked. Public opinion softened, and by the time of his death, Rockefeller was remembered mostly as a generous philanthropist.

While Lee is considered by many to be the father of modern public relations, a contemporary of his, the flamboyant Edward Bernays, engineered some of the most far-reaching, successful, and outlandish PR campaigns in history. He was derided by many of his colleagues for his brazen tactics and tireless self-promotion, but there is no doubt he was proud of his work. Bernays kept almost all of the notes and documents that crossed his desk during a career that spanned eighty years, and he left more than eight hundred boxes of them to the Library of Congress, with the stipulation that they be made public only after his death.[5]

Bernays was said to think of himself as a "unique counselor" to organizations, someone who melded the influence of the media with the science of psychology. He is generally credited with coining the term "public relations counselor," which he used in his 1923 book, *Crystallizing Public Opinion*, the first book devoted to PR. He also taught the first class on public relations, at New York University in 1923. Bernays's skill with the media was the result of dogged work and innate talent, but his bent toward psychology was grounded in family—he was a nephew of Sigmund Freud, with whom he had a close relationship.

Bernays was sophisticated and, like Lee, well educated. He was born in Vienna in 1891 but grew up in New York City. His first job after graduating from Cornell was as a writer and editor for a medical journal. From there, he ventured to Broadway, where he was a press agent for a variety of productions and celebrities, including Russian ballet dancer Vaslav Nijinsky and Italian tenor Enrico Caruso.

The Roaring Twenties brought profitability to a large number of new or revitalized industries, including one that became a mainstay for Bernays: tobacco. The American Tobacco Company, manufacturer of Lucky Strike, the United States' fastest-growing cigarette brand, was one of his biggest clients. Bernays said later that the head of American Tobacco, George Washington Hill, was determined to expand his company by tapping the potential of the women's market. The percentage of women smokers had been rising since the Great War, but Hill wanted to pick up the pace. According to Bernays, it was Hill's idea to tout cigarettes as a low-calorie alternative to sweets.

Bernays orchestrated a campaign that equated cigarettes with slenderness, grace, and beauty. He enlisted third-party "experts" to warn against the adverse effects of desserts, in terms of both weight gain and tooth decay, and to declare that cigarettes were a great alternative and could do everything from clean your teeth to make you a better dancer. Bernays's staff even distributed menus that substituted cigarettes for desserts. Despite some backlash against Bernays and American Tobacco, Hill wrote to Bernays in December 1928 that the company's revenue was up by thirty-two million dollars that year and that sales of Lucky Strikes had increased more than those of all other brands combined.

Even so, Hill was still dissatisfied with the number of women smokers in 1929. His insistence that Bernays come up with a way to get women to smoke outdoors as well as indoors led to the PR man's most notorious staged event. Bernays obtained a list of New York City debutantes and invited each one to join other women demonstrating their support for the equality of the sexes by walking together in the city's Easter Parade on Fifth Avenue in 1929. Additional women were recruited through ads signed by prominent local advocates of women's rights. All the information stressed that as the women walked, they would light symbols of equality, their "torches of freedom"—cigarettes.

The carefully scripted event went without a hitch, despite fewer than a dozen women showing up. Photos of them—defiant, stylishly dressed female smokers making their way through the parade—were published across the country, and several "torches of freedom" marches followed in support. Women, in other words, took the bait and proclaimed their determination to squelch the old taboo against smoking as the start of a movement to establish their equality with men.

Recounting the event in *The Father of Spin*, author Larry Tye explains that Bernays almost always failed to point out that the campaign was funded by American Tobacco and that letters used to recruit participants never mentioned the source of the idea or the funding behind it. Ironically, Bernays, who lived to be 103, supposedly never smoked and once admitted that he did not like the taste of tobacco. "I prefer chocolate," he said.[6]

DECIPHERING PEACETIME PROPAGANDA

Bernays, better than anyone, demonstrated the successful adaptation of wartime PR and propaganda techniques for use in postwar and depression-era America, but these increasingly brazen efforts did not go unnoticed or unopposed.

Between 1937 and 1942, the Institute for Propaganda Analysis worked to expose domestic propaganda that the group considered a potential threat to American democracy. Although the name itself sounds like propaganda, the IPA was a legitimate organization, created "to teach people how to think rather than what to think." Made up mostly of social scientists and journalists, it published newsletters that "examined and exposed manipulative practices by advertisers, businesses, governments, and other organizations" and sponsored related programs within high schools, colleges, and civic groups. It had no political affiliation.

Although the group was disbanded during World War II (reportedly because of the wartime conundrum of examining not only enemy propaganda but Allied tactics as well), the IPA left a notable legacy: its list of eight "Rhetorical Tricks" used by propagandists remains strikingly relevant to PR today. It includes the following basic propaganda/PR ploys:

1. **Fear** Organizations with the most to lose are most likely to resort to fearmongering. Their information may mention the loss of jobs, a threat to public health, or a general decline in social values, standard of living, or individual rights. It may also vilify a specific cause or even a specific person in order to create the desired point of view.

2. **Glittering generalities** This approach arouses strong, positive emotions by using words and phrases like "democracy," "patriotism," and "American way of life." Virtually all types of organizations use the tactic to create support for themselves, but when combined with negative messaging, the implications can be insidious.

3. **Testimonials** Celebrities or recognized experts are frequently recruited or hired to provide testimonials about a product, cause, company, organization, or candidate. Good examples are the photos of famous athletes on Wheaties boxes and the endorsements of causes of all stripes (from animal rights to the right to own guns) by actors and musicians.

4. **Name-calling** Blatant insults can be a very effective public relations tool. The organization doing the name-calling may associate the target of the insults with a negative or unpopular

cause or person. Defending against name-calling can be difficult. Negative terms tend to stick, even if they are undeserved.

5. **Plain folks** Anytime a business executive poses with rank-and-file employees or customers, he or she is claiming to be "of the people." The same goes for politicians who attempt to identify themselves with their constituents; with every election cycle come the candidates who claim to be "Washington outsiders" even if they've been in office for years. Being identified with "plain folks" is both good business and good politics, but it raises the possibility of being labeled a hypocrite.

6. **Euphemisms** PR practitioners often select words that obscure the real meaning of actions or concepts. The tactic is sometimes called "doublespeak." For instance, an employee may be "transitioned" rather than "fired," and a "lie" may be called a "strategic misinterpretation."

7. **Bandwagon** The overriding bandwagon message is that everyone else is doing or supporting this—and you should, too. Opinion polls can create the impression that a large percentage of people are on the bandwagon, but poll results may reflect only a designated sliver of the population, and they can be shaped in advance by structuring questions to trigger an expected response.

8. **Transfer** Similar to testimonials, the transfer approach involves the approval of a respected individual or organization. The IPA described transfer as "a device by which the propagandist carries over the authority, sanction, and prestige of something we respect and revere to something he would have us accept."[7]

ETHICS? WELL, SOMETIMES

As I said, PR has also been used to great and positive effect for deserving individuals, organizations, and causes. When skilled PR professionals do their jobs ethically, society benefits. For example, initiatives to end disease and poverty, to find missing children, to promote literacy, and to reduce violence have benefited from well-designed and well-executed PR campaigns.

But PR tactics are also used to create subversive front groups, discredit legitimate individuals or organizations, spread false information, distort the truth, and instill fear. In the recent debates on health care reform, we saw PR used to leverage fear so effectively that it convinced a good number of people to take positions contrary to their own best interests.

While most practitioners adhere to basic standards, there is no law to prevent any of them from violating the ethics of the profession, although scores of PR organizations have adopted guidelines for proper behavior. PRSA points to its own voluntary Code of Ethics as the industry standard. "Ethical practice is the most important obligation of a PRSA member," states the preamble. To that end, the code itself emphasizes the importance of honesty, expertise, and accountability in conjunction with loyalty to and advocacy on behalf of clients. PRSA members sign a pledge that espouses "truth, accuracy, fairness and responsibility."

PRSA boasted more than twenty-one thousand members in 2010 (I'm one of them), plus an additional ten thousand members in its student organization, the Public Relations Student Society of America.[8] Any member can report a violation of the code, and the organization has a process for reviewing and evaluating such reports. But there is no ongoing monitoring of the standards among members, and the concept of ethics can be easily lost in the enthusiasm of working for a high-paying client.

One of the most notorious examples occurred in 1986, when Anthony Franco, president of PRSA at the time, resigned after the SEC charged him with insider trading of a client's stock.[9] Today, the group's board of directors reserves the right to bar or oust individuals who violate the Code of Ethics, but the code's "emphasis on enforcement" was formally eliminated in 2000.

Many other practitioners have made headlines when caught carrying out campaigns that were based at least in part on deceptive PR practice. One of the most publicized cases, largely because it involved the nation's largest PR agency and also its biggest public company, took place in 2006.

The year was a rough one for Wal-Mart. The gargantuan retailer was being widely criticized for paying workers low wages and not offering health benefits to many of them, so it turned to its PR agency, the industry-leading Edelman, to improve its image. As one of the most media-savvy agencies around, Edelman chose to use the burgeoning niche of social networking as a tool to enhance the public perception of Wal-Mart. Renowned for touting ethics as a touchstone of the PR business, Edelman proceeded to leap over the ethical line by using a practice called "astroturfing." The term means creating a false grass-roots movement so that a carefully crafted campaign or event seems to be happening spontaneously.

In March 2006, the *New York Times* and *Wall Street Journal* reported that Edelman was recruiting bloggers to publish pro-Wal-Mart information. Marshall Manson, a senior account supervisor with Edelman at the time, provided regular e-mails to the bloggers, who used the material at their own discretion, with or without attribution.[10]

In October of that year, Edelman (a firm I once hired to do some work for CIGNA) took another public hit on behalf of Wal-Mart when BusinessWeek.com exposed an ostensibly independent blog titled Wal-Marting Across America as an Edelman project. This fake blog (or "flog") was presented as a middle-class adventure, with a couple—Laura and Jim—chronicling their cross-country RV trip by stopping in Wal-Mart parking lots along the way. Many of the people Laura and Jim encountered (and interviewed) were Wal-Mart employees, uniformly happy with their job and their employer. BusinessWeek.com blew the cover by outing the two as freelancers. Money for the RV, the gas, and fees for Laura and Jim came from a Wal-Mart-funded group called Working Families for Wal-Mart.

Edelman's CEO, Richard Edelman, confessed in his own blog that the agency had violated its stated ethical standards by setting up the "Laura and Jim" road show. However, he stressed that he was not personally involved in the project, which lasted only a few weeks before being busted. Wal-Mart, meanwhile, disavowed any connection to the debacle.[11]

Although there was speculation at the time that Edelman might suffer because of the bad publicity, there has been little, if any, negative long-term consequence. In fact, *Adweek* named Edelman the 2009 PR Agency of the Year, and *Advertising Age* declared the agency to be the top PR firm of the decade. The *Advertising Age* announcement, issued on December 14, 2009, included this statement: "The only major hiccup these past 10 years was the Wal-Mart Across America blog snafu back in 2006."[12]

PR also crosses the line when trying to repress or create doubt about information that could be harmful to a client. In 1994, for example, a whistle-blower from Ketchum PR disclosed that the firm had attempted to discredit a book called *Diet for a Poisoned Planet*. Because the book contained information about the dangers in some foods and might damage Ketchum's clients in the food industry, the agency took extreme steps to undermine the author's book tour. Ketchum, the sixth-largest PR firm in the United States at the time, obtained a copy of the author's schedule and arranged for someone to follow his itinerary and counteract his statements at every stop. In addition to spreading negative information about the author, Ketchum also used its influence to have as many of his major interviews canceled as possible.[13]

Edward Bernays, the master manipulator himself, was also forced to face the potentially horrific consequences of his own PR tactics. In 1928, he wrote in *Propaganda*, perhaps the most famous of his books, about the necessity of manipulating public opinion: "We are governed, our minds molded, our tastes formed, our ideas suggested, largely by men we have never heard of. This is a logical result of the way in which our democratic society is organized. Vast numbers of human beings must cooperate in this manner if they are to live together as a smoothly functioning society."[14]

In 1933, according to his autobiography, a foreign correspondent who had just returned from Germany dined at Bernays's home. The guest told Bernays, the son of Jewish parents, that he had recently been in the home of Joseph Goebbels, Adolf Hitler's Reich minister of propaganda in the rising Nazi regime, and had noticed at least one of Bernays's books in Goebbels's library. The guest told Bernays that Goebbels was using the book as a foundation for a campaign against Jews.[15]

Even more disturbing, the führer himself discussed manipulation of public opinion in his book, *Mein Kampf*, in terms that could be used by one of today's PR counselors. Hitler wrote, "The receptivity of the great masses is very limited, their intelligence is small, but their power of forgetting is enormous. In consequence of these facts, all effective propaganda must be limited to a very few points and must harp on these in slogans until the last member of the public understands what you want him to understand by your slogan. As soon as you sacrifice this slogan and try to be many-sided, the effect will piddle away, for the crowd can neither digest nor retain the material offered."[16]

Bernays fretted publicly about ethics in PR later in his life. Looking back, he said that had he known the dangers of tobacco, he would not have accepted the American Tobacco account. "No reputable public relations organization would today accept a cigarette account since their cancer-causing effects have been proven," he wrote in 1986.[17] Also late in life, Bernays appealed to PRSA to police its ranks, arguing that circumstances allowed unethical behavior without any sanctions, legal or otherwise. "There are no standards," he said. "This sad situation makes it possible for anyone, regardless of education or ethics, to use the term 'public relations' to describe his or her function."[18]

LIKE WATCHING SAUSAGE BEING MADE— OR WORSE

The best public relations is invisible. While it's easy to spot advertising— the stuff that blatantly urges you to go buy something—PR subtly convinces you to change the way you think. Advertising urges you to do something now; PR is patient. Advertisers pay for the time and space devoted to their messages. Good PR usually gets free media space because it is presented as unbiased information.

Dedicated PR pros consider their profession a science, grounded in research, strategy, and evaluation. They're trained to craft effective messages and to place them in media that will most effectively reach their target audiences. Good PR leaves little to chance. Good PR is about control.

Large companies typically have large PR departments, in which individuals may be assigned to particular media or to segments of the firm. Structure is tight, and jobs are well-defined. Big firms, as well as many small ones, also use independent PR agencies, periodically or on an ongoing basis. Media relations specialists, whether company or agency, deal with news-media representatives, planting stories, spinning information to a client's advantage, and choosing the best media to reach the target audiences.

News releases explaining what happened at an event are commonly written before the event takes place. Corporate executives go through "media training" to prepare them for speaking directly to reporters. Mock press conferences are held to give execs practice. PR staffers prepare a list of expected questions and appropriate answers for them in advance of media interviews. Few politicians and virtually no business executives write their own speeches. All good executives, like politicians, are taught the cardinal rule: Stay on message.

For many years, I was the designated media relations person, the company's public presence, the mouthpiece for management. Mine was the face presented to the media whenever my company was in the spotlight, voluntarily or otherwise. Never—not once—did I answer questions or make statements on behalf of my employer without knowing in advance what I would say.

PR people are good at manipulating news media because they understand them. A large number of practitioners are former reporters—like Lee and Bernays (and me)—who know what kinds of stories get attention, as well as who decides what gets coverage and what doesn't. Conversely, news outlets are increasingly dependent on public relations departments and agencies for content. As budgets drop, especially at newspapers, there are fewer reporters and fewer resources for investigative journalism. Canned information from companies is used "as is" more frequently, often without fact-checking.

In addition, PR people cultivate reporters, ostensibly for friendship or mutual benefit, but more realistically for manipulation. And in a disturbing trend, reporters can increasingly be cowed by powerful public relations reps because PR controls access to major news-makers in both business and government. I should know. For years, I was the gatekeeper to the CEO and other top executives at CIGNA. No reporter got to them except through me. I decided who had access and on what terms.

Unexpected things happen, of course, but PR people have a plan for that, too: crisis management—always in place, ready to be tweaked to fit individual circumstances, and set to be implemented on a moment's notice. A major negative event will kick the process into gear, and if the plan is executed well, the public will eventually perceive nothing more than a company that responded quickly and honestly to a problem.

The 1982 Tylenol tragedy is a textbook example. The entire country was stunned by the news that seven people in Chicago had died after consuming cyanide-laced capsules of Tylenol. Johnson & Johnson, the maker of Tylenol, immediately worked with news media to notify the public of the potential danger. The company recalled Tylenol from all store shelves voluntarily. Behind the scenes, Johnson & Johnson's CEO formed a strategy committee to determine the best way to prevent further deaths, and he worked extensively with his public relations staff and an outside agency to plan for the reintroduction of Tylenol in tamper-resistant packaging.

The result: 90 percent of the polled public said they did not hold the company responsible for the incident, and Tylenol sales began to skyrocket shortly after the product was back in stores. The *Washington Post* praised the firm for its performance, noting in an editorial, "Johnson & Johnson has effectively demonstrated how a major business ought to handle a disaster."[19] The poisoning case was never solved.

In 1982, communications were primitive by today's standards. There was no public Internet, no Twitter, and no cell phones. Newspapers, magazines, radio, and television were the only mass media. Confronting a crisis in today's era of media overload is much more complex. Not only do companies have more opportunities to reach and influence their target audiences, but they also face greater and far more immediate criticism when they get things wrong.

A recent example is Toyota's handling of its 2010 quality control debacle, in which more than eight million vehicles worldwide were recalled, resulting in a drop of more than 20 percent in the value of Toyota stock. The company's early response was slow, passive, insufficient, even insulting. Toyota was lambasted for ignoring customer complaints and denying safety problems that reportedly led to more than fifteen deaths. Bloggers, not to mention late-night talk shows, had a field day bashing Toyota. Other car manufacturers, even those facing recalls of their own, basked in relief that it was the world's largest carmaker taking the heat and losing business . . . to them.

Watching the Toyota crisis play out reminded me of the many times I'd been in charge of crisis communications throughout my career. When a crisis comes calling, PR people go into damage control mode. I was a fireman as well as a spinmeister, working to keep my clients and employers' reputations from going down in flames when something bad happened.

Fortunately, I didn't have to wear my firefighter's hat every day. Because of my role as chief spokesman, I spent much of my time fielding questions from reporters or schmoozing with them. I was not always writing press releases or pitching story ideas. In fact, I made it clear to the company's business and marketing people that I would not pitch a story that I knew had no news value. Instead, I worked hard to make sure that reporters saw me as a good and credible source of information about the insurance industry and trends in health care. Senior executives knew that I had developed good relationships with key reporters, and that I was able to influence what they wrote about CIGNA, which is one reason I survived several regime changes and restructurings during my fifteen years at the company.

With years of practice, I had learned how to respond with a pithy remark if I wanted to be quoted and how to "baffle them with bullshit" if I didn't. Soon after I joined the company, a colleague gave me a framed E. B. White quote as an inside joke: "Be obscure clearly." I became a master at doing just that.

To be a credible source for reporters, I had to spend a lot of time on conference calls and in meetings with business leaders to stay on top of what was going on. I started every Monday with three back-to-back calls and meetings, the first with the company's lobbyists in Washington, the second with my boss, and the third with the other PR people in the company, which I called our "news desk" call. The purpose of the call was to keep each other apprised of media inquiries, pitches, and anything else we were working on for our internal "clients." (We operated as an in-house PR agency, so we called the business people we worked with our clients.)

My staff and I also compiled a news summary every morning of all significant stories about CIGNA and the insurance industry that had appeared in the media over the preceding twenty-four hours. I never wanted any of our executives to be out of the loop or blindsided because they hadn't seen an important story.

In addition, we wrote speeches for the CEO and other top executives and cranked out a constant stream of documents and publications, ranging from media statements and position papers to the company's annual report to shareholders.

As chief gatekeeper, I decided who was worthy of interviewing our CEO and how much time they got with him once I'd determined the access to be in the company's best interest. I never let in a reporter I didn't know or have some sense of trust in. I prepared an extensive memo for the CEO each time, telling him what questions to expect and the talking points he should use regardless of what he was asked. I also included biographical information about the reporter and attached several recent stories he or she had written. I always sat in on the interviews so I could cut them short if they were going south.

I stayed in the CEO's good graces because I never left anything to chance. I planned ahead, and I kept my cool whenever the inevitable crises arose.

So, with that kind of résumé, I certainly didn't expect that a simple trip back home to the mountains of east Tennessee would make me lose this cool—and actually begin rethinking my life's path as a spinmeister.

But it did.

CHAPTER IV

Remote Area Medical in Wise County, Virginia

O N July 18, 2007, a little more than a month after the U.S. premiere of *Sicko*, former U.S. senator John Edwards (D-N.C.) made a campaign stop a few miles from where I grew up, in the southern Appalachians. A leading contender for the Democratic presidential nomination at that time, Edwards had decided to stop in Wise County, Virginia, as part of his three-day, eighteen-hundred-mile Road to One America tour, whose aim was to draw attention to the increasing number of Americans living in poverty.

I never would have known that Edwards was in the area if I hadn't taken a few days off to visit my folks in Kingsport, Tennessee. I learned from the media there that Edwards was coming to Wise County because it was the site of a big health fair at the county's fairgrounds. "Edwards Stops in Wise County to Address Health Care Concerns," said the front-page headline of my hometown newspaper, the *Kingsport Times-News*. The paper made the fair sound like such a big deal—thousands of people from as far away as Ohio and Alabama were expected to attend—that I decided to go check it out.

I was attracted particularly because one of my responsibilities was to keep CIGNA's CEO and other top executives up to speed on what the leading candidates were saying about health care reform. Another responsibility was to draft position papers and devise talking points on topics pertaining to health care reform—and one of the stickiest topics, of course, was the uninsured. In fact, I had been working for weeks on a paper that would eventually spell out CIGNA's stance on the main problems affecting the American health care system and how lawmakers should go about fixing them. I had presented a draft of this paper to CIGNA's fifteen-member Public Policy Council—headed by CEO Ed Hanway—shortly before my visit home.

Hanway had originally instructed me to focus the paper on the problems of the uninsured, but he later changed his mind, deciding that he wanted it to be more about what he referred to as "the real cost-drivers of health care." He said it was still OK to mention the uninsured in the paper, but not so prominently on the front page. He also said that when I did write about the uninsured, I should emphasize the fact that most Americans had health care coverage—and not the fact that forty-five million didn't.

Since Hanway also chaired AHIP's Strategic Communications Committee, it was clear that his new instructions to me represented the approach the industry would be taking when the reform debate heated up. The goal would be to divert the public's and the media's attention from the uninsured and toward problems the insurers could insist were beyond their control. The industry's spin, in other words, was going to be something like this: Health care costs are out of control because new treatments and technologies are more expensive than ever, the population is getting older and sicker, too many people are seeking care they don't really need, and health care providers are all too willing to provide this care that people don't need.

Knowing that Democratic candidates for president would likely blame insurance companies for both rising costs and the rising number of uninsured people, Hanway and the CEOs of other big companies (who controlled AHIP's purse strings) had begun plans for a multi-million-dollar public relations and advertising campaign to try to reframe the debate, shifting the focus away from their companies. The name of this effort would be the Campaign for an American Solution.

One of the CEOs' least favorite candidates was Edwards, who seemed to be intent on becoming the leading insurance company basher.

Sure enough, Edwards lived up to his reputation that day in Wise County. "[Lack of] access to affordable health care is a shameful aspect of a nation that should do much better by its citizens," the candidate said during his brief stop. "How can we live with this in America?"

AMERICA JOINS THE THIRD WORLD

While Edwards talked with reporters, there were hundreds of unconnected volunteers at work around him and in the background—converting the Wise County Fairgrounds into what over the following three days would become the site of Remote Area Medical's eighth annual expedition to the area.

Remote Area Medical (RAM, for short) is a Knoxville-based organization founded twenty-five years ago by, of all people, Stan Brock, co-star of *Mutual of Omaha's Wild Kingdom*, a popular and long-running TV show that premiered in the early 1960s. I didn't know anything about RAM until I read about it in the Kingsport paper on that visit.

Now seventy-four, Brock has an interesting life story—he left his family and private school behind in England when he was seventeen to seek adventure in the wilderness. He found it in Guyana, a small country then called British Guiana on the northeast coast of South America, between Venezuela and Brazil. For fifteen years, he lived and worked among the Wapishana and other Amerindian tribes there, helping them drive cattle through the country's savannas and rain forests to steamships that delivered them downriver to be sold at market. On one of these trips, Brock was badly injured when thrown from his horse. He needed medical care, but he was forced to heal without it—the nearest doctor being twenty-six days away on foot. Brock was aware that he lived in a remote area, of course, but he hadn't realized until then just how remote.

It was during his years in Guyana that Brock was discovered by the *Wild Kingdom* crew, while they were filming in the region, which eventually led to his TV career.

But before he left Guyana for his new and better-paying job, Brock saw several other health disasters unfold, like whole tribes nearly wiped out by illnesses that could have been easily treated back home in England. So he vowed that one day he would find a way to deliver basic medical aid to the people there and to people in other remote parts of the world. He made good on that pledge years later when he founded RAM, which began flying doctors and medical supplies from the United States to villages where he used to live. This outreach eventually morphed into a highly mobile relief force of doctors, dentists, optometrists, nurses, and medical technicians who volunteer their time to treat hundreds of patients a day under some of the worst conditions imaginable—not only in South America but also in Africa and Asia and, more recently, Haiti.

Brock first visited Knoxville when he was invited to appear there at a fund-raiser for the Knoxville Zoo soon after he left *Wild Kingdom*. He liked the area and the people so much that he decided to relocate there from Florida and make Knoxville the headquarters for his new venture.

It never occurred to Brock when he started RAM that most of his expeditions would eventually be to communities in the United States. But it soon became apparent to him that millions of Americans don't have much better access to care—or at least to care they can afford— than people in third world countries.

It started for him one day in the early 1990s when he got a call from a social worker in one of the poorest places in the country: Hancock County, Tennessee, about seventy miles north of Knoxville. The county had just lost its only dentist, and the only hospital had recently closed because of budget problems. The social worker had heard of RAM and asked Brock if he had ever thought about doing an expedition in the United States—and if so, would he please start in Hancock County?

"I was told that dental care was one of the biggest needs," Brock said, "so we loaded up a pickup truck with some old dental chairs and took a couple of dentists up there." It wasn't long before he was also taking doctors and medical equipment.

The word began to spread, and Brock was soon getting calls from other communities in the area. One of them was Mountain City, the small town in Johnson County at the northeastern tip of Tennessee where my parents were born and raised and where I had spent the first six years of my life.

Hancock, Johnson, and Wise counties have a lot in common. They are among the most remote counties in the southern Appalachians, miles from the nearest interstate highway, and doctors and medical facilities are far from plentiful. Few residents ever make it to college, and few employers are big enough to offer health care benefits.

Brock still does expeditions in Hancock County, but he stopped going to Johnson County a few years ago when his partners there decided to devote their resources elsewhere. Shortly before that, he was introduced to Wise County when a Catholic nun—who had operated a traveling medical clinic since 1980 in some of the most isolated counties in southwest Virginia—met Brock in Mountain City and persuaded him to take an expedition to Wise. He agreed, and the first Wise County expedition took place in 2000. The demand became so great that Brock decided to continue his partnership with Sister Bernie Kenny and her Health Wagon.

Sister Bernie turned over the reins of the Health Wagon in 2005 to nurse-practitioner Teresa Gardner, her longtime associate, and Gardner became the driving force behind the Wise County event, now one of the largest RAM expeditions in the United States. Over three days in July 2009, seventeen hundred volunteers contributed twenty thousand hours of time and more than $1.5 million in care, while recording more than seven thousand patient contacts.

A LIFE-CHANGING TRIP TO THE MOUNTAINS

The news coverage of John Edwards's visit to the 2007 RAM expedition led me to borrow my dad's old car and drive the fifty miles from Kingsport to Wise early on Friday, July 20. I'd seen a lot of health fairs over the years, some even sponsored by my employers, but never one as big or as comprehensive as the one I'd read about in the *Times-News*. My curiosity was in high gear.

The Wise County Fairgrounds covers several acres and is host to some of the area's biggest and most popular events. The month before, it had hosted the Mountain People's Music Fair. A few weeks after the RAM expedition, it would be the site of the Virginia-Kentucky District Fair & Horse Show.

When I arrived at about eight A.M., the parking lot was already jam-packed with cars and trucks. State troopers were directing traffic on all the nearby roads, and dozens of volunteers were trying to help latecomers find places to park.

On its Web site, RAM advises people attending the Wise County expedition to come early and come prepared: "Plan for long lines. It is not uncommon for as many as 500+ people to be in line at the start of a clinic day. Remember to bring food, water and an umbrella, and expect long delays."

Many people, I learned later, arrive the day before and spend the night in their car or a tent. On the day I was there, the first day of the clinic, eight hundred people had lined up before dawn to be sure they could get in when the gates opened at five thirty A.M.

Because the fairgrounds are walled in at the entrance, I couldn't see what was going on inside as I walked up to the registration desk. There were several volunteers there, but they didn't seem to be especially busy. Except for the sounds of car tires on the gravel in the parking lot as people came and went, it was eerily quiet.

Nothing prepared me for what I saw when I walked through the gates. The contrast to the calm on the outer side of the wall was stunning. The scene inside was surreal. I felt as if I'd stepped into a movie set or a war zone. Hundreds of people, many of them soaking wet from the rain that had been falling all morning, were waiting in lines that stretched out of view. As I walked around, I noticed that some of those lines led to barns and cinder block buildings with row after row of animal stalls, where doctors and nurses were treating patients. Other people were being treated by dentists under open-sided tents. Many were lying on gurneys on rain-soaked pavement. Except for curtains serving as makeshift doors on the animal stalls, there was little privacy. And unlike health fairs I had seen in shopping centers and malls, this was a real clinic. Dentists were pulling teeth and filling cavities, optometrists were examining eyes for glaucoma and cataracts, doctors and nurses were doing Pap smears and mammograms, surgeons were cutting out skin cancers, and gastroenterologists were conducting sigmoidoscopies. Huge amounts of medications were being dispensed.

I didn't realize until later that the *New York Times* had sent a reporter and a photographer to the Wise County expedition. The headline on the eight-page spread in the paper's magazine summed it up well: "Patients Without Borders: What Do the Uninsured in America Do When They Need Health Care? Some Turn to a Volunteer Medical Group That Was Set Up to Provide Free Services in Third World Countries."

In the article, Brock noted that despite the expedition's three-day span, hundreds of people are turned away every year, and that the medical needs of the people who come for free care far outstrip what the volunteers can provide. He said, "There comes a point where the doctors say: 'Hey, I gotta go. It's Sunday evening, and I have to go to work tomorrow.'"

Brock estimates that by 2010 about twenty-six thousand volunteers for RAM had treated more than three hundred thousand patients during six hundred expeditions in the United States and abroad. Because the need for the services that RAM and its volunteers provide shows no sign of abating, Brock is trying to raise one million dollars to expand the organization's capabilities. He hopes to use the money from RAM's "Reach Across America" campaign to, among other things, buy and operate another airplane to fly volunteers "anywhere we're invited." One of the planes RAM currently uses, which Brock himself flies, is a DC-3 used by the U.S. Air Force in Europe during World War II.

As I took in the scene at the Wise County Fairgrounds, I realized that the folks in those lines and animal stalls could have been my relatives or my parents' neighbors. I could tell from their faces that they were people with whom I shared cultural roots, but who—for whatever reason—simply hadn't had the good fortune to land a high-paying job and a cushy office in a Philadelphia skyscraper. Quite unexpectedly, this spur-of-the-moment outing was starting to feel personal and even spiritual—and I didn't consider myself to be much of a spiritual kind of guy. It was clear to me at that moment that I was having an epiphany.

As I noted earlier, one of the responsibilities of that high-paying job I had back in Philadelphia—a responsibility made all the more urgent as the health care reform debate intensified—was to try to convince the public that the problem of the uninsured was not so much of a problem at all. The real purpose of that document I had been working on for weeks was to sell the idea that insurers were the true good guys in the U.S. health care system, that they were blameless when it came to rising premiums, and that the growing number of people without coverage was not as serious a problem as many people believed.

I had used the U.S. Census Bureau's reports on the uninsured, which the bureau updates annually, as the primary source of my information for the document. These reports are a treasure trove of statistics.

While I was working on my document, a book that I had been assigned to read in college many years before came to mind: *How to Lie with Statistics.*[1] The teacher hadn't asked us to read it to learn how to deceive people, but rather to learn to recognize the tricks that people and organizations often use to mislead by slicing and dicing numbers in certain ways.

Using 2006 Census Bureau data on health care coverage, I selected statistics I felt would lead people to question whether the problem of the uninsured was as big as reform advocates claimed. One such statistic was that more than 40 percent of the uninsured are young adults, many of whom probably believe that the risk of illness or injury is too low to justify the cost of insurance. Another was that more than 35 percent earn at least $50,000 (and consequently should be able to afford insurance). Yet another was that more than 20 percent are not even U.S. citizens.

The clear implication of the statistics I chose was that most of the uninsured people in this country were simply shirking their personal responsibility to buy coverage or shouldn't be here in the first place. If the government would just force them to buy coverage from private insurance companies or enroll in a public program—or deport them— the problem would largely go away.

I knew that what I was writing would likely wind up in the hands of friendly members of Congress and conservative pundits who would use the statistics as part of their propaganda campaigns to keep comprehensive reform from ever happening. I also knew that the statistic about a fifth of the uninsured being noncitizens would really rile them. I knew that many people would interpret that to mean that they were all illegal aliens, while in fact many of those noncitizens were people in the United States legally, on either study or temporary work permits, who could not get or afford coverage. Many were performing jobs that U.S. employers had hired them to do because there were not enough Americans interested in or capable of doing them.

Probably the one sentence in the Kingsport newspaper story that had compelled me to go to Wise in the first place was this one: "Two-thirds of the people who avail themselves of free health services at the annual RAM event have jobs but no health insurance." I did not really believe (as I was implying in the paper I was writing) that the folks attending the expedition were lazy, irresponsible bums. So I think I went to prove to myself that they really were hardworking people who either couldn't get insurance or couldn't afford it. I knew—although I didn't mention it in my paper—that the median household income in the United States was just slightly more than $50,000.[2] (In Wise County, it was just a little more than $26,000. In Johnson County, it was just $23,000.) Another important fact I didn't include in the paper was that the average cost of a family health insurance policy had risen to $12,106 in 2007. (By 2009, it had increased to $13,375.[3] The average income for a minimum-wage employee, meanwhile, was just $11,500 in 2009.)[4]

Most of the employers in the southern Appalachians are small businesses—the Wise County Web site lists only four private employers in the county with more than sixty employees—and, as elsewhere in the country, more and more of them are dropping coverage for their employees because of the exorbitant rate increases that insurance companies have been imposing in recent years. Thousands of small businesses across the country have stopped offering coverage to their employees over the past fifteen years, in many cases because profit-driven health insurers have "purged" them from their rolls.

SCALES BEGAN FALLING FROM MY EYES

Among the many reasons I finally left my job at CIGNA was that with each promotion, I got a better understanding of how insurers get rid of enrollees they don't want—the very people who need insurance—when they become a drain on profits. I could no longer in good conscience continue serving as a spokesman for an industry whose practices, I had come to realize, were swelling the ranks of the uninsured. Instead of being part of the solution to the crisis of the uninsured, as I had long tried to convince the public they were, insurers had become the leading cause of the crisis.

To help meet Wall Street's relentless profit expectations, the for-profit insurers that now dominate the industry routinely dump policyholders who are less profitable or who get sick. Insurers use several techniques to cull the sick from their rolls. One is policy rescission, the common but until recently largely unknown practice in the insurance industry of retroactively canceling policyholders with large medical bills. *Los Angeles Times* reporter Lisa Girion stumbled upon the practice as she was gathering information for a story about a lawsuit that had been filed on behalf of a self-employed scrap metal hauler who was suing Blue Cross of California for canceling his policy retroactively after he underwent a procedure to clear blockages in his arteries. The insurer (now called Anthem Blue Cross) claimed that when he'd applied for coverage, he'd failed to disclose that he had suffered from heartburn in the past. After canceling his policy, Blue Cross told him he would be responsible for paying $130,000 in medical bills.

Girion wrote later that when her story appeared, in March 2006, "my in-basket overflowed with emails from readers telling me the same thing had happened to them or someone they knew. They all said their insurers had accused them of lying on their applications after they incurred significant medical bills." Her stories on the practice prompted state insurance regulators and a congressional panel to launch investigations. They discovered that insurers scour the medical records of policyholders who start filing expensive claims, looking for reasons to cancel their policies.

The congressional investigation into the rescission practices of just three insurers revealed that they had canceled nearly twenty thousand policies retroactively over a five-year period after going back to look at the original applications of policyholders who were undergoing expensive care. Rescinding those policies enabled the companies to avoid paying three hundred million dollars in claims. If the investigation had been broadened to include more insurers and had covered a longer period of time, Congress undoubtedly would have discovered that the practice is far more widespread.

In May 2010, Reuters reported that WellPoint, the parent company of Anthem Blue Cross, "singled out women with breast cancer for aggressive investigation with the intent of cancelling their insurance." WellPoint acknowledged that it had rescinded a number of breast cancer patients' policies but denied that the women had been singled out. Reuters stood by its story. It noted that WellPoint was one of the three companies investigated by Congress (UnitedHealth Group and Assurant Health were the others) and that the investigation had revealed that WellPoint alone had profited by more than $128 million from canceling policies retroactively, a figure that investigators believed "might be largely understated because the company refused to provide information about cancellations by several subsidiaries."

When members of Congress asked executives of the three companies if they would end the practice of rescission, they said they would not. That's because dumping even a small number of enrollees can have a big, positive effect on the bottom line. (It literally took an act of Congress to force the companies to change their policies. It will become illegal under the Patient Protection and Affordable Care Act of 2010, except in cases involving intentional fraud.)

As I mentioned previously, another way insurers get rid of enrollees they no longer want is to dump small businesses when some of their employees' medical claims turn out to be greater than the insurance companies' underwriters expected.

All it takes is one illness or accident among employees at a small business to prompt an insurance company to hike the next year's premiums so high that the employer has to cut benefits, shop for another carrier, or stop offering coverage altogether—leaving workers uninsured. This is the practice known in the industry as purging. The purging of less profitable accounts through intentional rate increases helps explain why the number of small businesses offering coverage to their employees has fallen from 61 percent in 1993 to 38 percent in 2009, according to the National Small Business Association.[5]

CIGNA got some very unwelcome publicity a few years ago when it tried to impose such a hefty rate increase on one customer, the Entertainment Industry Group Insurance Trust, that some family-plan premiums would have exceeded forty-four thousand dollars a year.

Jacking rates up so high that customers don't renew their policies is common. Aetna was so aggressive in getting rid of accounts it no longer wanted after a string of acquisitions in the 1990s that it shed eight million enrollees over the course of a few years. The *Wall Street Journal* reported in 2004 that Aetna had spent more than twenty million dollars to install new technology that enabled it "to identify and dump unprofitable corporate accounts."[6] Aetna's investors rewarded the company by running up the stock price. Reuter's investigation of WellPoint revealed that the insurer used a "fuzzy logic" program to help identify policies to cancel. Health Net acknowledged that it had paid bonuses to employees who found policies the company later rescinded.

Insurers take these actions because they want to get rid of risk—policyholders who are costing them more money in claims than they had anticipated. For-profit companies are most aggressive in doing this because of the constant pressure from Wall Street to meet their earnings expectations. After acknowledging in a 2008 conference call with financial analysts that her company had spent more on medical care during the previous three months than the analysts had expected, WellPoint's CEO, Angela Braly, promised that in the future, "we will not sacrifice profitability for membership." WellPoint and other insurers have shown, however, that they are perfectly willing to sacrifice their members for profits.

LET THEM EAT CAKE—AND SEND THEM
TO ANIMAL STALLS WHEN THEY GET SICK

When I went back to my job at CIGNA's corporate headquarters after my trip to Wise County, my mind was in turmoil. I was trying to process what I had seen. I talked to some of my colleagues and even showed them pictures I had taken at the expedition. I was having a very hard time finishing the health care reform document I had been assigned.

The power of my experience in Wise County really hit home a couple of weeks later as I was boarding one of the two private jets CIGNA uses to fly executives around the country. I flew on those jets several times a year. With conference tables, video screens, leather seats, and deep carpet, they make first class on a commercial airliner look shabby. As usual, on this flight, which was taking me to a meeting in Connecticut, a uniformed attendant brought me lunch on a gold-rimmed plate and handed me gold-plated flatware with which to eat it.

My thoughts turned immediately to the people I had seen being treated in animal stalls just days earlier.

A few months later, I saw an article in *Architectural Digest* with a headline reading, "Romancing the Stone: In the Hills of Eastern Pennsylvania Rises a Prototypical French Farmhouse." Amid a sequence of elegant photos, it described a twenty-four-room mansion inspired by "ancient stones of *la France profonde*" and featuring "an impossibly French" kitchen with a "white-walnut winery sorting table" and a separate "grandchildren's cottage" of stone columns imported from Europe.

The magazine didn't disclose the name of the retired executive for whom this mansion was built, but it was common knowledge in the executive suite at CIGNA who lived there. It was the company's former chairman and CEO, Wilson Taylor, whose salary in 2000, his last year with the company, was twenty-four million dollars—which doesn't include the additional millions he reaped from stock options and deferred compensation.

When I read that article and saw the stunning pictures of Taylor's new place, it became clear to me, in ways that it hadn't before, that people enrolled in CIGNA's insurance plans had actually helped pay for that twenty-four-room stone manse with its seventeenth-century Spanish columns and its impossibly French kitchen.

Furthermore, I could now see clearly, those people in Wise County would not have had to stand in line in the rain for hours to get care in animal stalls if so much of the money Americans spend for health care didn't wind up in the pockets of insurance company executives and their Wall Street masters.

CHAPTER V

Health Care History, Reform, and Failure

UNLIKE developed countries that took deliberate action at their highest levels to create the national health care systems they currently enjoy, America largely forfeited the development of its system to private, financially motivated interests from the very beginning. The result is that universal health care is available today in every industrialized nation except one—ours. (It's also available in many developing countries.)

As another consequence, these powerful special interests became so entrenched in our nation over the years that almost no president was able to overcome their organized opposition to reform until now, the sole exception being Lyndon Johnson—whose administration, in a historical breakthrough, saw the 1965 creation of two government-run programs, Medicare and Medicaid. The reform bill that Congress passed in 2010 is potentially far-reaching, but lawmakers gave up on the idea of creating a new government program—the public option—because of opposition from the insurance industry.

Before I detail for you how the health insurance industry and its allies waged their ongoing fearmongering and misleading campaigns against recent reform, let's pause to look back in history. And while doing so, let's chant the old axiom: The more things change, the more they stay the same.

There is little in the newest rounds of deceptive PR and advertising efforts that is different from the strategies of antireform campaigns in America's past, and this includes the very language and the illusion of spontaneous "grassroots" uprisings, which have been employed by the special interests of every era.

A vivid example is Ronald Reagan's participation in the American Medical Association's famous propaganda campaign against early Medicare legislation in 1961. The AMA cloaked this effort, called Operation Coffeecup, in a low-key shroud fronted by the association's own Women's Auxiliary, whose members invited their friends and colleagues to about three thousand neighborhood kaffeeklatsches across America. Once confined and regaled with hospitality, guests were entertained further by their hostesses, who played a professionally cut vinyl LP titled "Ronald Reagan Speaks Out Against SOCIALIZED MEDICINE."

In an eleven-minute impassioned plea on the disc, Reagan railed against Medicare as "socialism" and argued that it was the "foot in the door" to a totalitarian takeover of everything we knew. After doctors were subdued, he warned his mostly female listeners, big government would eventually come after America's children: "And pretty soon your son won't decide, when he's in school, where he will go or what he will do for a living. He will wait for the government to tell him where he will go to work and what he will do!"

He urged his coffee-sipping listeners to write their local congressmen to oppose any government intrusion into the free-market health care system and concluded, "Write those letters now. Call your friends and tell them to write them. If you don't, this program, I promise you, will pass just as surely as the sun will come up tomorrow. And behind it will come other federal programs that will invade every area of freedom as we have known it in this country, until, one day . . . we will awake to find that we have socialism. And if you don't do this, and if I don't do it, one of these days, you and I are going to spend our sunset years telling our children, and our children's children, what it once was like in America when men were free."[1]

Although it lobbied openly in Washington and elsewhere, the AMA made no effort to claim this campaign. Instead, it made every effort to keep the sponsorship under wraps in an extremely slick PR ploy for its day. The AMA wives and other recipients of the LP were not allowed to broadcast it commercially, and they were encouraged to make the entire letter-writing campaign resemble a gigantic ground-swell of antisocialist sentiment. There were conflicting claims later about the number of letters that resulted, but nobody disputes that the result was substantial.

Reagan was eventually "outed" that summer by the mainstream media for his partnership with the AMA, and the credibility of the overall campaign (which featured "antisocialism rallies" in several states) was called into question, but Reagan's effort served as a tremendous personal boost to the then B movie actor and General Electric TV host's political career. Some Reagan biographers credit this episode as the beginning of his ascent to the White House.

Although Medicare's proponents eventually won, another thing is certain: The Reagan LP previewed the exact talking point language used to provoke fear over the subsequent five decades about "the sun-set of America" if any real health care reform should pass at the federal level. Sarah Palin even quoted from Reagan's disc during her Republi-can nomination acceptance speech in 2008.

It shouldn't be surprising how effectively this "paranoid style" continues to work in American politics. Pulitzer Prize–winning histo-rian Richard Hofstadter coined this term in his 1964 book, *The Para-noid Style in American Politics*, which attempted to explain the McCarthy era. The message from our contemporary right wing is the same as the one Hofstadter wrote about nearly half a century ago. The view, he said, is that "old American virtues have . . . been eaten away by cosmopolitans and intellectuals; the old competitive capital-ism has been gradually undermined by socialistic and communistic schemers; the old national security and independence have been de-stroyed by treasonous plots, having as their most powerful agents not

merely outsiders and foreigners as of old but major statesmen who are
at the very centers of American power. Their predecessors had discovered conspiracies; the modern radical right finds conspiracy to be be-
trayal from on high. Important changes may also be traced to the
effects of the mass media."

HEALTH CARE IS DIFFERENT IN ISOLATION

There is a strong element of historic reality supporting this contra-
dictory American thinking. While Europe had had nothing but entrenched monarchies and/or strongly centralized, warmongering (or
cowering) governments, America was coping with a totally opposite
set of problems, most of them derived from its strongly decentralized
government—namely slavery, secession, civil war, reconstruction, and
unbridled expansionism—when the abstract idea of national health
care reared its head in the late nineteenth century.

Actually, as an infant republic, the United States had earlier mim-
icked European nations by starting one of the world's first government
health programs. President John Adams signed a bill in 1798 establishing the Marine Hospital Service, a federal network designed to care for
seamen, who paid twenty cents a month to belong and have access to a
group of hospitals in U.S. seaports. The MHS eventually evolved into
today's Public Health Service, a major part of the Department of
Health and Human Services, headed by the surgeon general.

But if you weren't a seaman, organized health care simply
didn't exist for you during the next century—except for a few sporadic
experiments that dot the history books, mostly as footnotes. For example, there was Massachusetts Health Insurance of Boston, organized in 1847 and usually credited as being our first "sickness"
insurance; a French mutual-aid society (la Société Française de
Bienfaisance Mutuelle) that in 1853 began offering prepaid hospital
care in San Francisco, a system closely resembling that of HMOs today; and, in the decades following the Civil War, a number of mining,

industrial, and railroad companies that began providing on-site doctors for workers who prepaid with deductions from their paychecks.[2]

World health care changed abruptly and forever in 1883 when one of history's most unlikely people, Otto von Bismarck, founder of the German Empire and known as the Iron Chancellor, ordained the world's first "compulsory sickness insurance" as part of his political effort to develop a strong working class as the foundation of a strong Germany. Although he is remembered in this country mostly as the strong militarist and nationalist that he was, Bismarck also went on to create the world's first social security retirement system in 1889—arguing that "people who know they are cared for are the best building blocks for a strong nation."

The irony today of detractors calling national health care "socialist" must certainly have Bismarck spinning in his grave. It is no paradox that he and those who followed in his footsteps established European health systems as extremely conservative antisocialists— they were catering to the working classes as leverage against their joining true socialist and labor movements of the day. Strong conservative governments in Europe called this "turning benevolence into power"—a strategy generally credited with creating the social welfare measures that actually kept Communism from becoming a dominant force.

Similar health care systems followed in Austria in 1888 and in Hungary in 1891. After their success was evident, another round of reform brought compulsory sickness insurance to Norway in 1909, Serbia and England in 1911, Russia in 1912, and the Netherlands in 1913. France and Italy adopted different approaches, subsidizing mutual-benefit societies that workers formed among themselves. Others, like Sweden, Denmark, and Switzerland, chose instead to give strong financial assistance to voluntary funds, beginning in 1891.[3]

Because of its uniquely decentralized government and lack of any need (yet) for antisocialist political paranoia, the United States simply rode out this period of health care history, no one pushing the agenda. Instead, another American phenomenon, for-profit life insurance, gained ground, with a boom in the sale of weekly-premium policies that provided lump payments at death, which could be used to pay for final care and burial. Exploiting the fear of a "pauper's burial," these policies were sold by aggressive people who also collected the cash premiums—ten, fifteen, or twenty-five cents a week—to fuel a highly profitable industry that boasted a staggering 60 percent administrative cost (yes, only 40 percent of premiums actually went to benefits). Thus was a new American personage created, the insurance agent. Metropolitan Life and Prudential Insurance Company led an explosion so great that by 1911 Americans were spending about as much ($183 million) for this product as Germany did for its health system that year.[4]

AMERICA'S FIRST "EUROPEAN INVASION"

It wasn't until 1906 that the first national noises were made in the United States for actual health insurance. That year, the American Association for Labor Legislation (AALL) was established at the University of Wisconsin by a group of academic reformers that included prominent economists of the Progressive Era. Among their chief supporters on the political side was President Theodore Roosevelt, who often paraphrased Bismarck by saying that "no country could be strong whose people were sick and poor." But Roosevelt had his political agenda full with reforming basic capitalism in the Progressive mold—a far bigger necessity at that time—and he never got around to health care before leaving office in 1909, thus becoming the first president (of many) in that category.

Health insurance advocates got a major boost when Roosevelt came out of retirement, bolted from the Republican Party, and ran as a candidate for the Bull Moose Party in the election of 1912. Many historians say it was the high-water mark for Progressivism, arguing that Roosevelt's defeat by the conservative Democrat Woodrow Wilson left a void in the kind of presidential leadership needed to enact social welfare programs. Perhaps so, but AALL tried to carry out an ambitious reform strategy—and, in so doing, became the first reform victim of its own political naïveté, not to mention the first reform casualty of the same fearmongering propaganda that has been echoing ever since.

AALL and its allies from the Progressive Era did have one major textbook success with their efforts during the years of the Wilson administration and World War I. They lifted the abstract idea of universal health care to an unprecedented level of popular acceptance in this country and provoked a feeling by many citizens that it was imminent—only to be savagely frustrated and thwarted. This familiar cycle would be repeated four more times during the twentieth century— the next time, during Franklin Roosevelt's New Deal era; after that, under President Harry Truman; in the early 1970s, when Watergate killed more than a presidency; and lastly, during the Clinton health-plan debacle of 1993–94.

All five efforts emerged from different political circumstances. But if all five were recast as *Law & Order* or *CSI: Miami* episodes, despite there being five different victims, five different sets of fingerprints, and five different murder weapons left at the scene, the motive would be the same. And the only possible conclusion would be that they were all "done in" by the same "perp": America's free-market health care system, which walked away scot-free each time.

Because it was the first victim, the AALL effort is worthy of study. In short, the group comprised about three thousand reform-minded members, mostly upper- or upper-middle-class leaders in their communities or regions, giving AALL considerable influence. As an "elitist organization," AALL was anything but liberal. In fact, most of its members were vigorous opponents of Eugene Debs, leader of the Socialist Party, who was on a tear at the moment. AALL members sought to neutralize these Socialist Party inroads by using "scientific methods" to aid the working classes while also eliminating the abuses of capitalism—loosely imitating the earlier conservative, nationalistic European successes.[5]

As part of the Progressive Era, and enlightened by their own pragmatic backgrounds, AALL members recognized from the outset that the strongly decentralized government of the United States required an approach radically different from the social welfare systems in Europe. It would be more difficult to install as well, because all programs would have to be legislated at state and local levels rather than at the federal level, as on the other side of the Atlantic. President Wilson's general opposition to any federalized social legislation further mandated this route.

The first national AALL campaign was for states to legislate that employers form government-run pools to insure their workers against industrial accidents—providing "workmen's compensation." This campaign met with very little resistance and a great deal of enthusiasm. Thirty-three states eventually passed such laws. Encouraged and inspired by this and other local successes (and even buoyed by Roosevelt's impact on the 1912 election), AALL upped the ante and set its sights on its major Progressive goal: government health care at state levels in America.[6]

An AALL national conference in 1913 eventually led to formal input from the AMA, and in 1914 the two groups formed an actual partnership of sorts that led to the drafting in 1915 of a bill that was thought to be acceptable to all. Limited to the working classes, the proposed bill would have provided coverage for physicians, nurses, and hospitals, plus sick pay, maternity benefits, and a fifty-dollar death benefit for burial costs. Hopes were at their highest.

But 1917 saw the house of cards come tumbling down. Big labor, spearheaded by Samuel Gompers, denounced compulsory health insurance as an unnecessary, paternalistic reform. State and local medical societies objected to the AMA's support of the legislation, which led to the national group's denying that it had ever sponsored it in the first place. And—surprise, surprise—also joining the opposition were the for-profit life insurance companies, which vociferously objected to the legislation's "intrusion" into their market, despite the fact that none of them offered health insurance.

This sudden, unforeseen groundswell of opposition probably would have been enough. But another major event, the U.S. entry into World War I in April 1917, engulfed the entire debate in a fierce anti-German fever. Opponents labeled the effort "un-American" and the "Prussian menace" and claimed it was part of a plot designed by German dictator Kaiser Wilhelm II "the same year he started plotting and preparing to conquer the world." Prudential Insurance executive Frederick Hoffman called the reformers' proposal for a European-like compulsory insurance program a "German plot."[7]

California was the only state to go ahead with a public referendum, in 1918, but it was vigorously opposed by the state's physicians, who were joined by the major life insurers' group, led by Prudential and Metropolitan, and the Pharmaceutical Manufacturers' Association, which financed a campaign to galvanize public opposition.

The referendum became the first overt effort by special interests in the United States to defeat health care by using propaganda—and by then the Russian Revolution had occurred, so the by-now-familiar epithets "Bolshevik" and "Communist" joined "Hun" and "Prussian" in pamphlets as descriptions of people who supported the plan, which lost overwhelmingly at the ballot box.

THE FREE-MARKET "SOLUTION" CONTINUES

The Red scare continued after the end of the war and brought public hysteria to new levels in America. Triggered by a wave of inflation, a series of violent labor strikes, race riots, lynchings, and other forms of vigilante justice, the United States entered a period of political unrest that changed little throughout the 1920s. In this panicky climate, further proposals for "socialist" public health care reform simply did not happen.

Free-market, prepaid health insurance began creeping into existence, though, with the introduction of company group plans, like one offered by Montgomery Ward & Company in 1910, and labor union plans, like one offered by the International Ladies Garment Workers Union in 1913. Such plans covered less than 2 percent of the workforce by 1929, when the nation's first real public prepaid-hospitalization plan was unveiled in Dallas.

The focus of the plan was narrow, specifically a single institution—the nonprofit Baylor University Hospital—where the administrator, Dr. Justin Ford Kimball, devised a strategy to deal with the hospital's mounting expenses. His idea was to have groups of local residents, beginning with Dallas teachers, pay fifty cents a month and receive up to twenty-one days of hospital care—if needed—during any year. Called the Kimball Plan, it made everybody happy, subscribers and cash-strapped hospital officials alike. Other nonprofit hospitals quickly began mimicking it, but all these early plans mandated that enrollees use only the hospital initiating each scheme.

"Free choice" plans that allowed subscribers to choose their own "participating" nonprofit hospital when ill soon began popping up. Some of these plans were killed quickly in states that saw this as selling insurance without a license, infringing on the free market. But this, in turn, prompted the American Hospital Association to lobby states to permit the sale of hospital insurance by nonprofit corporations, like hospitals—an idea approved first in New York in 1934 and then by thirty-five other states during the next eleven years.

Eventually, these tax-exempt efforts were united under a common name, Blue Cross, and a common trade group, the Blue Cross Association (later renamed the Blue Cross and Blue Shield Association),[8] which by 1945 had about two thirds of the nation's health insurance market locked up, in what undoubtedly is by far the biggest consumer-driven success story in America's history of open-market health insurance. The fact that it was accomplished by government-shielded nonprofits doesn't deter today's talking point propagandists from extolling its "free-market" approach.

Unfortunately, in 1929 something bigger than the birth of what would become Blue Cross also happened: the Wall Street crash and the Great Depression.

Although serious health care issues went unaddressed at any political level in the 1920s, the process of thinking about them didn't stop. A productive result was the Committee on the Costs of Medical Care, founded in 1927 and led by Dr. Ray Lyman Wilbur (president of Stanford University, a former AMA president, and a future secretary of the interior) to attempt the first-ever serious study of U.S. health care and how to change or improve it.

Made up of fifty high-level economists, physicians, and public health specialists, the CCMC, in a report it released before disbanding in 1932, called for far-reaching changes in the organization and financing of American medicine, although stopping short of asking for compulsory insurance. Its primary recommendations were for medical practices to organize with hospitals as their focus rather than solo practitioners; for public health services to be extended; for group payment for medical care to be established through taxation, private health insurance, or both; and for there to be large-scale planning for and coordination of the nation's health services.

Although these proposals may seem rather reasonable and tame—even conservative—in today's world, they were deemed totally unacceptable by a majority of physicians at the time. The AMA, now ever vigilant, denounced them as "an incitement to revolution." Other health providers attacked them as an attempt to "institutionalize" and, of course, "socialize" American medicine, which up to that point had been a highly individualistic, largely self-regulated affair. Instead of illuminating a well-reasoned path to the future, the CCMC's 1932 report helped underscore the sharp divide between doctors and the rest of society that still echoes today.[9]

It was into this cauldron that Franklin Roosevelt tumbled that year by being elected president to deal with the greatest economic crash in the nation's history. A quarter of the population was unemployed, banks were collapsing, industries were bankrupt, there was panic in the streets, and Roosevelt assumed a national presidency that gave him little executive power to do much but watch the suffering. Understandably (and supported by everyone but the radical right), Roosevelt immediately began legislating ways to obtain and centralize the executive power needed for someone in his position to deal with these staggering issues. Also understandably, health care just wasn't on that list—yet.

SOCIAL SECURITY, YES; HEALTH CARE, NO

The first two years of Roosevelt's New Deal were a whirlwind of activity that led to the establishment of a great many agencies to combat the depression, many of them stopgap or emergency measures but all of them reflective of a never-before-seen level of executive energy coming from an extremely activist central government. Coupled with his Fireside Chats over the radio, Roosevelt's actions served to lift America's spirits, while changing the very nature of government and public policy. Eventually, during one of his famous chats, he said, "One of the duties of the state is that of caring for those of its citizens who find themselves the victims of such adverse circumstances as makes them unable to obtain even the necessities for mere existence without the aid of others. That responsibility is recognized by every civilized nation . . . To these unfortunate citizens aid must be extended by government—not as a matter of charity but as a matter of social duty."

It was in this vein—citing the vast inadequacies of state-run programs—that Roosevelt appointed a Committee on Economic Security (CES) in June 1934. Chaired by Secretary of Labor Frances Perkins, it was to study all forms of national "social insurance" and to make recommendations by the end of the year. Although Roosevelt said in a

June 8 address to Congress that he was particularly interested in old-age and unemployment insurance, he opened the door for explorations of accident insurance, retirement annuities, survivor's insurance, family endowments, maternity benefits, crop insurance—and health insurance.

The AMA again mobilized at once, eventually calling an emergency meeting of its House of Delegates (only the second in its history), which denounced any effort to "socialize" medicine by establishing prepayment plans and taking health care decisions out of the hands of physicians. The siege had begun, with AMA members and staff bombarding members of Congress with letters, postcards, and phone calls decrying any form of compulsory health insurance. Edwin Witte, executive director of the CES, recalled that the committee was "at once subjected to misrepresentation and vilification."[10]

The pressure continued unabated, publicly and privately, for a year—and included the president's own personal physician lobbying Eleanor Roosevelt.[11] The president responded by appointing physicians to the CES and seeking a middle ground that would be acceptable— but the AMA would have none of it, and the pressure continued until an evening in June 1935, when Roosevelt privately concluded to his administration that it should proceed with a Social Security bill on its own merits, not risking its defeat by including health care provisions.

For the next seventy-five years, scholars would debate whether the president was unduly cautious about health insurance. But all sides agree that the decision was Roosevelt's alone—and no one will ever know what would have happened had he committed to battling personally for health insurance in the overall Social Security Act, which he signed into law on August 14, 1935—a major milestone for the nation on its own. The victory was so huge, in fact, that Roosevelt's administration was consumed with other political battles spawned during its enactment period. This and other depression-era legislation— coupled with the rise of Blue Cross–type insurance for companies and their workers (eventually endorsed by the AMA)—placed public health care on the back burner again.

In July 1938, a National Health Conference was held in Washington to bring together (some say for the first time ever) all the disparate interest groups—including doctors, unions, farmers, and civic leaders—to discuss the health needs of the nation at that point. The conference concluded with a series of recommendations that featured increased public health services in general, aid for the medically indigent, grants-in-aid for hospital construction, and grants to states to encourage (but not compel) statewide health insurance plans.

The AMA called another emergency session of its House of Delegates—but this time it adopted a more conciliatory position, opposing only any language that might result in compulsory insurance. Several discussions on the matter ensued at the White House before Roosevelt abandoned the issue for that election year—which turned out to be prophetic. A conservative resurgence at the 1938 polls, led by Dixiecrats and Republicans, made things "righter" in Washington and effectively put an end to New Deal legislation.[12]

Health care came up again with Roosevelt in the White House. The following year, Senator Robert Wagner (D-N.Y.), a personal friend of the president, introduced the National Health Act of 1939. Roosevelt never put his weight behind Wagner's legislation, although it was endorsed by big labor (it was opposed by the AMA), and it was still in committee on September 1—the day Germany invaded Poland.

For the second time in the life of many Americans, military action in Europe put an end to any real talk about national health insurance—except for tax exemptions allowed for health benefits so that companies could attract and maintain private-sector workers during the war years. Many employers took advantage of the exemptions, bolstering the non-profit Blue Cross–type coverages already in the market and leading to the uniquely American employer-based health insurance system.

Wagner's bill evolved and was reintroduced in 1943 as the Wagner-Murray-Dingell Bill, which would have funded compulsory national health insurance with a payroll tax. Opposition was overwhelming, with the AMA adopting a question it's been asking us ever since: "Do you want medical care for the sick to be provided by bureaucrats or doctors?" Although now just a footnote in history, the bill remains interesting because it was introduced and defeated in every congressional session for the next fourteen years.

TRUMAN'S EFFORT PLANTED THE SEEDS

In 1945, Roosevelt died, the war ended, and Harry S. Truman became the first president in the nation's history to openly endorse a single universal comprehensive health insurance plan. Mincing no words, Truman's first major peacetime address to Congress, in November 1945, stunningly laid out this agenda. Noting that during World War II, nearly five million Americans had been classified as unfit for military service for health reasons, and that another three million had been treated or discharged for physical or mental problems that had existed before their induction, Truman introduced bills in both the House and the Senate, telling Congress, "In the past, the benefits of modern medical science have not been enjoyed by our citizens with any degree of equality. Nor are they today. Nor will they be in the future—unless government is bold enough to do something about it. We should resolve now that the health of this nation is a national concern; that financial barriers in the way of attaining health shall be removed; that the health of all its citizens deserves the help of all the nation."[13]

Once again, the AMA issued its call to arms, this time using to its advantage the cold war to cast Truman's "socialized medicine" as an extension of feared Russian communistic control of the world. "[If this] Old World scourge is allowed to spread to our New World, [it will] jeopardize the health of our people and gravely endanger our freedom," shouted the AMA *Journal*.[14]

Heeding the AMA's call, Republicans in the House blocked the bill from even getting a hearing, and they were joined in this opposition nationally by the American Bar Association, the American Hospital

Association, and most of the nation's press—who parroted the AMA argument that the legislation would make doctors "slaves." Truman countered by pointing out that it allowed doctors to choose their own form of payment, but these words fell on deaf ears. The bills didn't advance in 1946—and furthermore, the Republicans used them as proof of Truman's "socialism" to tailor a GOP sweep back into control of Congress in that fall's elections.

Truman retaliated by making public health care part of his own reelection platform in 1948, which mortified the AMA and other opponents when the feisty Missourian staged one of the biggest upsets in election history, also leading the Democrats back into power on Capitol Hill. Thinking that Armageddon had arrived, the AMA assessed each member an additional twenty-five dollars, hired a public relations firm (Whitaker & Baxter), and mounted an anti-Truman campaign in 1949 that cost $1.5 million—the most ever spent on a lobbying effort in the United States at that time.[15]

Part of the PR effort was a poster and a pamphlet distributed to patients in doctors' waiting rooms across America that urged, "The Voluntary Way Is the American Way." Insurers and employers were also enlisted as allies to the campaign, with the AMA in return urging its own members to ask patients to purchase private, voluntary insurance to head off the attempt to enslave them. The U.S. Chamber of Commerce pitched in, printing a pamphlet, "You and Socialized Medicine," that urged member companies to endorse and purchase private group-insurance plans for their workers to eliminate any need for a public plan. Racist Southern politicians also joined the opposition by preaching at home that the dangers of "socialized" medicine included an end to racially segregated hospitals and the enforcement of staff privileges for black doctors. By the end of 1949, the nation had witnessed its first-ever all-out paranoid-propaganda blitz by the country's for-profit, free-market health care sector.[16]

But the crowning blow once again came from overseas, where in late 1949 the Soviet Union announced the establishment of a

Communist government in East Germany and Mao Tse-tung's Communist party established the People's Republic of China. Despite the now-raging cold war, Democrats retained control of Congress in the 1950 elections, but the GOP made enough gains to slam the brakes on any further effort by Truman to get national health insurance back on the agenda.

"I cautioned Congress against being frightened away from health insurance by the scare words 'socialized medicine,' which some people were bandying about. I wanted no part of socialized medicine, and I knew the American people did not," Truman wrote later in his memoirs. "I have had some stormy times as President and have engaged in some vigorous controversies. Democracy thrives on debate and political differences. But I had no patience with the reactionary selfish people and politicians who fought year after year every proposal we made to improve the people's health."[17]

The AMA's opposition to Truman, and its successful partnership with business and private-pay insurance companies, put into motion the market forces that eventually took control of American health care. Companies like General Motors, for example, began paying for health insurance and pensions for their workers in 1950, igniting a shift that continued for decades—eventually leading to the takeover of health care by large for-profit insurance providers. Union leaders like Walter Reuther of the United Auto Workers foresaw this outcome when he expressed relief that his own insurance was being covered but ruefully acknowledged that this was not the strongest solution possible, which would be a system that covered everybody and spread the costs to all.

And sure enough, commercial insurers soon began cherry-picking young and healthy premium-payers by offering them lower prices. An increasing number of large employers realized, too, that they could self-insure by cutting their own deals with insurance companies, thus no longer needing to belong to the broader nonprofits. By the end of the 1950s, insurers were "experience rating" firms to base premium charges on a company's usage of services. All of these forces produced a golden age for the idea of free-market insurance. By 1963, nearly 80 percent of Americans were employer insured, and health care costs had largely been contained by market conditions.

FINALLY, GOVERNMENT-RUN HEALTH CARE, BUT NOT FOR ALL

By the 1960s, though, the nation's elderly were an increasing problem for the free-market solution because of their health care demands. Company health plans with benefits to retirees—mostly through unions—suddenly had to jack up current workers' premiums in order to cover rising costs. The rest of the elderly, mostly poor and un-insured, were creating larger demands on state and local charity suppliers. The "success" of America's health care solution had dramatically showed its Achilles heel.

The earliest reaction came in 1958, when legislation was introduced that would cover hospital costs for people on Social Security. As expected, the AMA swung into action—employing the same paranoid attacks as before—but this time the debate did not evaporate. By concentrating their focus on problems of the aged, proponents eventually passed a bill, in 1960, called the Kerr-Mills Act, which provided states with federal grants to pay for health care for the elderly poor. However, only twenty-eight states signed on to the plan, and many of these didn't set aside enough state money to trigger the federal response—plus doctors and hospitals rejected payments because they were "below the prevailing rate."[18]

So, for the first time in the nation's history, a groundswell of au-thentic grassroots support for a tougher law began rising. By 1962, polls were showing that 69 percent of Americans favored such a measure—by now called Medicare—and President John F. Kennedy joined in the support, making it a legislative priority. The frightened AMA this time created a political action committee, AMPAC—which recruited the personal doctors of members of Congress to lobby against the effort—as well as running familiar newspaper, radio, and TV ads decrying Medicare as socialized medicine. The legislation lost by narrow votes in the first round (by only 52–48 in the Senate), which gave Kennedy encouragement to introduce it again the following year, when it was stalled in the House Ways and Means Committee, but by the narrow vote of 13–12.

Although it had stalled the Medicare bill, the AMA (for the first time ever) began losing some of its partners—notably the American Hospital Association and some of the now-powerful for-profit insurance companies, who agreed to the need for a government program to pay health costs for the elderly because it was affecting their own bottom lines. With support from big labor, too, and universal support from elderly Americans, the Medicare idea was gaining steam when, in November 1963, Kennedy was assassinated and Lyndon Johnson assumed the presidency.

Aided by the shock of Kennedy's death and the landslide victory of Johnson and the Democrats in 1964—much of it the result of Kennedy's unfulfilled domestic agenda, which LBJ had reframed as his own Great Society—Medicare was shoved across the finish line in 1965, though not before some final tweaks and compromises.

Realizing its losing position, the AMA lobbied for what it called Eldercare, an amplified version of the Kerr-Mills Act. Insurance companies, led by Aetna, pushed for another version, called Bettercare, which would provide federal money to be used for private health insurance premiums for the poor and elderly. In the final showdown, Wilbur Mills, House Ways and Means Committee chairman, combined all three ideas into the final Medicare bill, which he called his "three-layer cake": Part A, which covered hospitals; Part B, which covered doctors and was optional; and Medicaid, a separate program for the states. Prescription drugs were not covered, nor were eyeglasses, dentists, and long-term care, but the final bill emerged as the largest expansion of health care coverage in American history.

In a special homage to Truman, LBJ signed the bill on July 30, 1965, in Independence, Missouri, with Truman at his side.

Johnson said, "No longer will older Americans be denied the healing miracle of modern medicine. No longer will illness crush and destroy the savings that they have so carefully put away over a lifetime so that they might enjoy dignity in their later years. No longer will young families see their own incomes, and their own hopes, eaten away simply because they are carrying out their deep moral obligations to their parents, and to their uncles, and their aunts."[19]

MEDICARE DIDN'T TOTALLY SOLVE THE PROBLEM

The implementation of Medicare and Medicaid consumed enormous attention in government and the health care world for the next several years, but by 1970 growing health care costs and increased numbers of uninsured among the non-elderly renewed the debate about more drastic health care reform. It was President Richard Nixon who helped sound the alarm, saying, "We face a massive crisis in this area. Unless action is taken within the next two or three years . . . we will have a breakdown in our medical system." He was supported by the normally conservative media, including *BusinessWeek* and *Fortune* magazines, which had cover stories and special issues declaring that American medicine stood "on the brink of chaos." Polls also showed that 75 percent of American households agreed there was a "crisis."[20]

Senator Ted Kennedy (D-Mass.), chairman of the Senate Health Subcommittee, opened fire in 1971 with renewed promotion of national health insurance. Nixon responded with his own plan, which would mandate employer health coverage for all working Americans and would require employers offering traditional indemnity coverage to also offer a prepaid group plan called, for the first time, a health maintenance organization (HMO). By July of that year, there were twenty-two different bills in Congress—ranging from Kennedy's comprehensive single-payer plan to a complicated but conservative scheme called Medicredit, supported by the AMA. It was an amazing time in politics—hardly imaginable today, the period from 1970 to 1974 was vividly alive with proponents for changing a system they all deemed to be in collapse.[21]

But because of the number of proposals, and the constantly shifting political alliances, Congress took no action on any of them in 1971 or 1972, an election year. The only plan to find common ground and get passed in 1973 was Nixon's Health Maintenance Organization and Resources Development Act (HMO Act), which required companies with twenty-five or more employees to provide an HMO option.

Despite all the fervor, the result had been "cycling negative majorities" of adherents to each plan, with the result that none could get majority support. Kennedy and Mills eventually joined in a compromise bill that had the best potential, but (a) Mills was brought down by a sex scandal (remember Fannie Fox?), and (b) Nixon resigned after Watergate.

Recession, inflation, the loss in Vietnam, the Arab oil embargo, and eventually the Iranian hostage crisis dominated the rest of the 1970s, stifling attempts at further reform. That period was followed by the conservative Reagan years, during which Nixon-era HMO enrollment grew fourfold as private managed care plans flourished in their new environment. By 1991, even longtime advocates for national health insurance like the *New York Times* were suggesting that private managed care (rather than public policy) should continue leading the way.

But under the surface—waiting to boil over again—was the fact that millions of American families were going without health insurance and therefore not part of any managed care solution.

Something else was boiling, too, by the time Bill Clinton was elected to the White House in 1992: the dominance of a handful of for-profit insurance providers that had consolidated their control over the health care system even more successfully than the AMA.

The Reagan years produced no meaningful debate over health

care, but they produced several changes in response to employer concerns about selection bias and HMO pricing. In October 1988, Congress enacted some pro-business amendments to the HMO Act that
relaxed regulations of federally qualified HMOs, basically freeing employers to negotiate HMO rates and coverage more easily—and lifting
federal equal-contribution requirements for companies.

This political period, in fact, merely solidified the control of our
health care system in the hands of a very few large corporations under
the broad category of "managed care," which I'll explain further in the
next chapter.

With the large, for-profit insurance companies now firmly in control, Hillary Clinton came to Washington to crusade for reform.

And I wasn't far behind, working against her.

CHAPTER VI

Consumer-Driven Care

THERE have been no Remote Area Medical expeditions to Pequot Lakes, in central Minnesota, but if Stan Brock leads one there before all the provisions of the current national health care reform kick in, Tom and Katie Brennan and their five children might be first in line.

Like millions of Americans, the Brennans are finding out what it means to be underinsured—and how far the American system of financing health care has strayed from the original concept of insurance, which was to spread risk over a large pool of policyholders so that everyone, regardless of age or health, paid the same amount for coverage.

The Brennans are a two-income family—Tom is self-employed; Katie is a schoolteacher—but they can barely afford the ever-increasing premiums and out-of-pocket expenses under their so-called consumer-driven health plans.

Because the premium increases for family coverage by the local school district had been in the double digits for years—26 percent in one recent year alone—Katie dropped her family from that policy. "The cheapest family plan our school offers has an $858 monthly premium and an $11,000 deductible, which means nothing is covered until you exceed that amount," Katie said when I talked to her. "That's just too expensive for most schoolteachers. Only half of the eighty teachers are still on one of the district's insurance plans."

Katie is now enrolled in a plan through the district that covers only her, with $150 monthly premiums (the school district pays an additional $300) and a deductible of $5,000. Tom pays $450 a month for a $5,900-deductible policy he obtained on the individual market for himself and their children.

Even with that coverage, they had to fight their insurance company last year when their son Jack broke his arm. The fight was not to get the insurer to cover expenses related to the accident—the Brennans paid all the bills because the total expenses did not exceed $5,900—but merely to get credit for the money they paid toward the deductible.

"[The insurer] said we needed to provide proof that it was not a preexisting condition," Katie said. "This was a little ridiculous since he broke his arm in July and we had had coverage with this insurance company since February."

The Brennans are thinking now that they would be better off without insurance. They pay more than $7,000 a year in premiums and still have almost $11,000 in combined deductibles—and they have to pay the full cost of prescription drugs because medications are not covered under either of their policies.

"Because of the high deductibles, we still wind up paying for everything out of pocket," said Katie. "We now avoid going to the doctor. It is just too expensive. The cost of our premiums and out-of-pocket costs exceed our monthly mortgage payments. We do not take family vacations, and we drive older cars because our budget is so tight."

While most of the people who seek medical care at RAM's expeditions have jobs but no health insurance, a fast-growing percentage are people like Tom and Katie Brennan, who have insurance that doesn't come close to covering their medical expenses. According to a study by the Commonwealth Fund, the number of underinsured Americans reached twenty-five million in 2007—up 60 percent since

2003.[1] At that rate of growth, the fund anticipates, at least forty million Americans might be underinsured—despite the reform bill just enacted—when it does a follow-up study in 2011. The reform legislation will help by limiting maximum out-of-pocket expenses that an insurer can require, but for many Americans these deductibles will still be more than they can afford.

A consequence of underinsurance is that many people don't get the care they need. In a separate study by the Center for Studying Health System Change, covering the same years as the Commonwealth Fund survey, one in five Americans reported delaying or forgoing needed care in 2007, up from one in seven in 2003, in many cases because they were underinsured.

Middle-income families are especially hard-hit by this trend. *American Medical News* noted in a 2008 story about the two reports that middle-income insured Americans "are increasingly experiencing health care access difficulties that are more commonly associated with their lower-income counterparts and the uninsured."[2]

This rapid growth in the number of underinsured Americans is a consequence of the continuous shifting of health care costs—through high deductibles and coverage limitations—from insurance companies to their policyholders.

As an insurance industry PR executive, I had the responsibility of helping create the perception that the high-deductible and so-called limited-benefit plans that insurers and employers were forcing Americans into were consumer-friendly and essential weapons in the industry's battle against escalating health care costs. I was expected to hype these plans as part of a "consumerism" trend that was started by Americans who wanted more control over their health care and their health care dollars. To perpetuate the myth that Americans were clamoring for health insurance plans that required them to spend more of their own money for their medical care, my colleagues and I were expected to follow the lead of our CEO and industry marketing types and call these plans "consumer-driven."

"Consumerism is an inescapable trend," declared Ed Hanway, CIGNA's CEO, in November 2005 at the company's Consumerism Forum for Investors, held at the überexpensive Mandarin Oriental, the swanky Manhattan hotel in Columbus Circle overlooking Central Park. "Like a tidal wave, it's building in size and intensity . . . The crowd is chanting more: more choice, more control over health benefits, more quality and value, and consumers know that they have more at stake both financially and, most importantly, in terms of their own health."

MANAGED CARE: WHAT WAS THAT ALL ABOUT?

"Consumer-driven" plans started appearing in the early 2000s when it became clear that the techniques of managed care—the insurance industry's silver bullet of the 1990s—had not lived up to expectations. They might have, had the big for-profit insurers not done irreparable harm to this once-popular means of keeping people healthy at relatively little expense. By the time they were done with it, managed care companies (usually HMOs) were almost universally loathed.

The forerunner of managed care plans—which require enrollees to seek care from a limited network of health care providers in exchange for relatively low premiums and out-of-pocket expenses—came into existence in the late 1920s and enjoyed wide support for decades, although mostly in Western states. A doctor and Lebanese immigrant named Michael Shadid is generally credited with developing the first one, in Elk City, Oklahoma, in 1928. Members of the cooperative, mostly farmers and their families, paid a fixed monthly fee in exchange for care at Shadid's clinic. Soon, in California, Drs. Donald Ross and H. Clifford Loos established a prepaid plan for employees of the Los Angeles water department.

The idea caught on. Industrialist Henry Kaiser was so impressed with what Drs. Ross and Loos had accomplished that he set up a similar arrangement for his workers who were building a large aqueduct in Southern California. That plan was the forerunner of the Kaiser Permanente health system, which now serves more than eight million enrollees in several states. The Ross-Loos Medical Group also experienced steady growth, eventually including a hospital and nineteen clinics in Southern California.

It was not until the Nixon administration, however, that these prepaid plans started spreading eastward. As I mentioned earlier, Nixon put his support behind a bill that would encourage the creation of health maintenance organizations, the new name for the plans. The HMO bill attracted bipartisan support and became law in December 1973. The growth of HMOs was assured through a provision that required employers with twenty-five or more workers to offer an HMO plan if they also offered a traditional indemnity plan.

When the big indemnity insurance companies started losing customers to HMOs, they did what they had to do in order to survive: They began buying their new competitors. CIGNA was among the first of the big national multi-line insurers to get into the HMO business through a series of such acquisitions. One of the first was the Ross-Loos Medical Group, soon renamed the CIGNA Healthplan of California.

CIGNA and the other big insurers set out to convince their corporate customers that they could keep their employee-benefit budgets under control if they moved their workers out of traditional indemnity plans, which allowed workers and their families to get care from any doctor or hospital, and into HMOs, which paid only for care provided by doctors and hospitals in defined and limited networks. HMOs could save money in a way that indemnity fee-for-service plans could not, by negotiating favorable rates with health care providers they wanted in their networks and by refusing to pay for care given to their members by providers who were "out of network." Later permutations of managed care plans, like preferred provider organizations (PPOs), would provide some coverage for out-of-network care, although enrollees would be on the hook for higher coinsurance payments if they went to a non-network physician or hospital.

My first experience as a promoter of HMOs came in 1985 when I was hired by the Baptist Health System of East Tennessee to run its advertising and PR operations. Baptist had just recently launched its own HMO with a network of its own three hospitals in the Knoxville area and the doctors who admitted patients to them. Many of the hundreds of HMOs that sprang up as a result of the HMO Act were local plans established by hospitals like Baptist, which saw HMOs as a means to attract patients.

I had no trouble being an HMO promoter while at Baptist. My family and I liked our HMO's emphasis on preventive care and the fact that we had a primary care physician who would coordinate care with specialists should we ever need them. Just as important, we liked knowing that visits to doctors would never cost more than a $10 copayment—and that we would never have to file another claim.

Attitudes toward HMOs began to change for the worse, however, when the big for-profit insurers began to take over. These insurers knew that the more HMO members they had in a given market, the more leverage they would have over local doctors and hospitals. Not only could the insurers demand deep discounts from doctors once they acquired significant market share, but they could also influence—through their reimbursement policies and coverage guidelines—how the doctors practiced medicine.

One of the reasons membership in HMOs grew so rapidly in the 1990s was because insurers were remarkably successful in getting their big-employer customers to move their employees out of indemnity plans and into HMOs. As recently as 1994, according to the Employee Benefit Research Institute, traditional indemnity plans were still the most commonly offered type of employer-based health plan. Just three years later, only 15 percent of workers were still enrolled in indemnity plans. The forced "migration" of workers to the managed care world was stunningly swift and successful.

It didn't take long, though, for doctors to start pushing back against the HMOs' policies of providing lower payments for services and requiring doctors to follow strict care guidelines to even be paid, which they considered an inappropriate intrusion into their practice of medicine. In 2000, doctors joined a massive class action lawsuit against all of the big national and regional insurers, including CIGNA. The lawsuit contended, among other things, that HMOs used a software program designed specifically to cheat doctors out of millions of dollars. The suit was eventually settled out of court, although the managed care companies admitted no wrongdoing. As part of their settlements, CIGNA and the other insurers agreed to make significant changes in the way they paid physicians and to reimburse more than seven hundred thousand doctors for claims they had previously denied. CIGNA's settlement alone was valued at four hundred million dollars.

By then, HMO members had also begun their own rebellion. They didn't like being told which doctors and hospitals they could choose and—even worse—being forced out of the hospital before their doctors thought they were ready. As described in chapter 1, the front-page stories in 1996 about HMOs insisting on one-day hospital stays for mastectomies and deliveries touched off a massive public outcry. Hardly a week went by when I didn't get a call from a reporter with an HMO "horror story."

The reputation of HMOs would never recover. The public came to believe that instead of improving care, as insurers had promised, HMOs and other managed care plans had actually reduced the quality of care in the United States. They were finding that their doctors were spending less time with them during appointments because HMOs' limited networks meant that network doctors had to take on more patients and, consequently, had to see more patients during a given day than they had in the past. And they were finding that HMOs were forcing doctors to adhere to what many of them referred to as "cookie-cutter" guidelines in delivering patient care. If they didn't follow the guidelines—or take the time to prove to the HMOs why certain treatments were appropriate for certain patients—they wouldn't get paid.

In response to the backlash, big insurers launched a major effort in 1998 to put a positive spin on managed care. The companies banded together to finance a front group they named the Coalition for Affordable Quality Healthcare (CAQH). They then hired Goddard Claussen, the firm that created the "Harry and Louise" commercials to help sink the Clinton reform plan, and the Hawthorn Group, a PR firm, to develop a campaign to improve the image of managed care. Knowing that doctors were much better liked and respected than HMO executives, the consultants recruited physicians to appear in a series of ads and commercials to testify why they thought managed care was a good thing for their patients.

The insurers funneled six million dollars into the campaign to counter what CAQH called "misperceptions" about managed care generated by media reports. In its first press release, CAQH said its ads would emphasize the message that managed care "keeps people healthier because it focuses on preventive medicine and provides the same high quality care at lower cost than traditional insurance." The campaign, it said, "will remind people of why they like their HMOs . . . It provides the health care you want at a price you can afford."

Despite the millions spent on the campaign, it didn't really "move the needle," as the industry's pollsters said a little more than a year after its launch.

This was an especially difficult time to be a PR guy for an HMO. I learned to avoid telling people at Little League games and holiday parties what I did for a living. Just saying that I worked for CIGNA was often all it took to get an earful.

I was conflicted. On the one hand, I felt that HMOs were getting a bum rap in the media. It seemed as if every reporter felt an obligation to bash managed care. On the other hand, I was beginning to have doubts that I was on the side of the angels. Defending my company and the industry was beginning to take a toll on me psychologically.

For the first time, I started questioning whether for-profit insurers really did play a constructive role in our health care system, as I insisted publicly. But it was all self-talk. I never told anyone I was having doubts. I found that alcohol helped to keep those thoughts at bay, so I drank more than I ever had—although never at work—to keep from dealing with recurring thoughts that I had sold out.

As part of my rationalization, I told myself that at least I was occasionally able to make a positive difference in a few people's lives. One of my responsibilities, when a health-plan member complained to the media about a treatment or procedure that CIGNA had refused to cover, was to make sure the company's executives understood what the PR consequences could be if the company didn't pay. While medical directors always said they would never change a coverage decision based on what the media might or might not do, denials that attracted media attention were often reversed. Whenever that happened, I took some satisfaction in thinking that I might have helped save someone's life.

I came to realize that many of my fellow employees engaged in the same kind of self-talk to get through the day. They were good people who had families and needed to keep their jobs just as much as I needed to keep mine. We told ourselves that for every horror story we heard, there were many more success stories, many more cases in which CIGNA paid hundreds of thousands of dollars for urgently needed care. And, we reminded ourselves, the media cover the few big wrecks on the freeway, not the thousands of people who make it home safely every day. To remind CIGNA's customers of that, my staff and I began producing a newsletter called *Proof That's Positive*. It consisted of anecdotes about people whose health had been improved and whose lives had been saved because their insurance company— CIGNA—had been there for them in their time of need.

My newsletter didn't seem to move the needle any more than the CAQH campaign. The backlash from members and the unrelenting negative publicity eventually forced insurers to loosen some of their coverage guidelines and restrictions and to broaden their networks of providers. Employers, fed up with complaints from their workers, pressured insurers to design "mixed model" benefit plans, like PPOs, that allowed enrollees to go out of network if they wanted to.

There is no shortage of irony here. Insurance industry executives contended that if the government would just get out of the way and let the invisible hand of the market work, managed care plans would reduce the number of people without coverage, improve quality of care, and be a permanent solution to rising health care costs. The promise was that the techniques of managed care would make government intervention into the financing and delivery of care unnecessary.

The invisible hand did work, but the results were the exact opposite of what the insurance industry executives had promised. When the marketplace responded, insurers had to sacrifice many of the very techniques that had briefly enabled them to control costs.

Rather than admit responsibility for the failures, insurance executives pointed the finger of blame at their customers, the "consumers" of health care, and, of course, the providers of care. In introducing the concept of their new silver bullet—consumer-driven health care—insurance executives claimed that the "real drivers of health care costs" (one of my CEO's favorite expressions) were the people who sought care when they really didn't need it and the doctors and hospitals who were all too willing to provide this unnecessary care. Sure, the aging population and expensive new technology were also factors, but the main culprits were people who just didn't realize how expensive health care had become.

There was one "mistake" that insurers were more than willing to admit to making, and this was that they had been charging HMO members way too little. Those modest ten-dollar copayments that once had been the centerpiece of HMOs' marketing strategies actually made Americans irresponsible consumers of health care. "What didn't work in managed care was that we separated the consumption of care from the cost of care," Hanway said at the CIGNA Consumerism Forum. "People didn't care what things cost anymore."

Hanway, who left CIGNA in 2009 at age fifty-seven with a $111 million retirement package,[3] was a leader in what Yale University political science professor and author Jacob Hacker calls the "personal responsibility crusade"—a euphemism for pushing risks, and costs, formerly borne by institutions onto individual Americans.

In his 2006 book, *The Great Risk Shift*, Hacker wrote that consumerism was part of that crusade, which grew during the administration of George W. Bush when Washington was "abuzz with discussions of Social Security privatization, Medicare reform, Health Savings Accounts, and scores of exotic new tax breaks to encourage families to set up private accounts to deal with economic risks of their own."[4]

Hanway, who gave ten thousand dollars to the Republican National Committee in 2003 and hosted a fund-raiser for John McCain during his bid for the presidency in 2008, rarely missed an opportunity to connect with his new personal-responsibility spiel. "The concept of consumerism . . . engenders personal accountability," he told corporate-benefits managers in a 2004 speech in Washington.

Another leader of the crusade was John Rowe, former chairman and CEO of Aetna, who left with a golden parachute of his own. "We are giving people some skin in the game," Rowe told financial analysts in 2002. Having people put more "skin in the game," Hacker wrote, is what the personal-responsibility crusade is all about. And the crusade leaders are well-paid CEOs and politicians.

DRINKING THE KOOL-AID

Consumerism in health care actually started in 1996, when the Republican-led Congress passed legislation creating a pilot project to encourage Americans to open medical savings accounts. The response was underwhelming. The bill's sponsors had hoped that 750,000 people would open such accounts, but only about 100,000 ever did.

Then in 2002, the IRS gave a new lease on life to what insurers would soon market as "consumer-driven care" when it ruled that the personal-spending accounts associated with these plans (called health savings accounts, or HSAs) were tax-exempt. The effect of that ruling was to turn HSAs tied to high-deductible, "consumer-driven" plans into tax shelters for people who made enough money to sock some of it away every payday. Proponents of HSAs argued that by spending their own money for care instead of relying on an insurance company, people would become more prudent "shoppers" of health care.

During the recent debate on health care reform, Republicans in Congress and other allies of the insurance industry said that Congress should scrap the Democrats' reform legislation and start over. When President Obama asked Republicans during his February 2010 bipartisan summit on reform what ideas they had to solve the country's health care crisis, Senator John Barrasso of Wyoming said that Congress should do more to encourage people to set up HSAs, which by law can be used only with high-deductible plans.

"John," Obama replied, "members of Congress are in the top income brackets of this country, and health savings accounts, I think, can be a useful tool, but every study has shown that the people who use them are folks who've got a lot of disposable income. And the people that we're talking about don't."

Obama was right. Just about every credible study has concluded that high-deductible plans are best suited for relatively young and healthy people who have a few dollars left over after they pay their bills. For the rest of the population, they frequently turn out to be a very bad deal.

At a leadership retreat I attended a few years ago, a vice president of a large insurer was trying to explain the benefits of consumer-driven care to about one hundred of his colleagues who were hearing about their company's consumerism strategy for the first time. He was having a hard time convincing them that consumer-driven plans would be good for certain segments of the population.

He was peppered with questions about how the plans could be a good deal for people with chronic conditions and people who didn't have extra money to put in a savings account or otherwise meet high deductibles. After about thirty minutes of nonstop questions, he finally said, "Look, you're just going to have to drink the Kool-Aid."

That was the end of the Q&A.

HYPE THIS, HIDE THAT

Knowing that studies on the underinsured like the ones from the Commonwealth Fund and the Center for Studying Health System Change would slow—if not halt—the trend toward consumerism, the big insurers began churning out their own "store-bought studies" to counter reality. As head of corporate PR, I was expected to hype CIGNA's proprietary studies—so from the very first such study, in 2006, our objective was to create the impression that a vast majority of enrollees were saving money and leading healthier lives.

A February 2, 2006, news release we sent out claimed that CIGNA's analysis of 42,200 of the company's first-time users of consumer-driven health plans—who were compared with users of HMO and PPO plans—found that they "generated an 8 percent reduction in medical costs" and "made positive changes in their behavior," such as increasing their use of medications to treat chronic health care conditions.[5]

The release quoted Michael Showalter, CIGNA's head of consumerism, as saying, "These study results show that given greater choice and control, the right incentives and actionable decision support, CIGNA Choice Fund [a consumer-driven plan] members are becoming more involved in their health care and health care decision-making, while not compromising needed care."

This release, however, omitted important information that actually reinforced the studies it was seeking to refute. One thing not revealed in the release was that the CIGNA Choice Fund group was younger than the comparable HMO and PPO groups; another was that the CIGNA Choice Fund group had a 20 to 25 percent lower "illness burden." In other words, the CIGNA Choice Fund group was younger and healthier than the older, sicker people who had stayed in their HMOs and PPOs. (In fairness, this information was provided in the appendix to the study, on page 17, deep in the Study Methods section.)

And then, there was this: While the news release claimed that people who switched to a Choice Fund plan realized cost savings "across all categories, with the most pronounced savings occurring among medium and heavy users of care," a more detailed analysis on page 8 of the study showed that heavy users actually fared worse. A graph on that page showed that the heavy users of care in the Choice Fund plan (those with medical claims of eight thousand dollars or more per year) actually paid *more* out of pocket than if they had been in traditional plans.

Because a business communications staffer had written and disseminated the release (my corporate PR team and I didn't have to approve all of the business units' communications), I hadn't noticed these differences between the study and the news release until after it had been sent out. While this certainly wasn't the first time in my career that I had seen or been at least partially responsible for the selective disclosure of information to support a particular point of view, it was the first time I became concerned that my colleagues and I might have crossed what for me was an ethical line. I began to think about my days as a reporter, when I'd felt it was my duty to make sure that the stories I wrote were factual and honest. Had I become the antithesis of what I'd tried to be as a journalist?

It was at that moment that I realized how much was at stake with the industry's transition from managed care to consumerism. The business model based on managed care had failed, and the only way the insurers could continue to meet shareholders' expectations was to find a new way to avoid paying for health care. The means now available to them was to shift costs to policyholders.

From that point on, I was skeptical of all claims coming out of my industry about the appropriateness of consumer-driven plans for large segments of the population.

As for that news release, while it didn't get much media pickup, I knew it would influence reporters' thinking even if they didn't write about it. And that was part of the objective: to try to get the media to question the findings of studies like the one from the Common-wealth Fund. Not a single reporter called me with questions about the methodology of the CIGNA study or the apparent discrepancies.

I wasn't surprised. With cutbacks in newsrooms, there were fewer reporters covering the health insurance industry than in years past, and the ones who were left were often so busy that they had little time to probe. I was frequently amazed at how little media scrutiny there was of the industry and at how much my colleagues and I could get away with in dealing with reporters. More often than not, they were quite willing to settle for what we fed them, even if it was pabulum.

NO SOLUTION FOR PEOPLE WITH
LITTLE SKIN TO SPARE

A few weeks later, I was looking for external studies to bolster the claim being made by the Bush administration and industry executives that the growth of consumer-driven plans would lead to a steady re-duction in people without insurance. Instead of finding evidence that it would happen, however, I came across a report written by a highly regarded former financial analyst that completely debunked the no-tion.[6] The author, Roberta Goodman, had covered for-profit health insurance companies for Merrill Lynch before starting her own con-sulting business. She got right to the point: "Consumer-driven health care cannot resolve the problem of the uninsured."

Goodman noted that 65 percent of the uninsured had an income below 200 percent of the federal poverty level. Few of these people would be able to afford the premiums of even a low-cost consumer-driven plan, she said, let alone fund an HSA. She also pointed out an-other fact: A significant number of Americans lack access to coverage because they are "medically uninsurable," meaning that insurers refuse to sell them coverage at any price because of preexisting conditions. "Their costs would almost inevitably exceed high-deductible plan maximums, so any plan available to them would require extremely high premiums."

The sickest 10 percent of the population—including many of the medically uninsurable—generate two thirds of health expenditures in any given year, Goodman wrote. If given a choice of plans, these people would undoubtedly steer clear of consumer-driven ones. "While some [of them] might benefit from early intervention, care management and clinical pathways tools . . . their costs [would] rapidly reach out-of-pocket maximums, and *cost often plays little role in the decisions of those facing critical illness.*" (Emphasis added: Goodman's point is just common sense. When you're sick with a critical illness, shopping for a bargain is not a top priority or desire. So much for the theory that big savings can come from people being more prudent "shoppers" of care.)

So, despite the hype from the health insurance industry, consumer-driven plans that shift more of the cost of care to individuals and families are not the silver bullet that will make America's health care system more efficient and equitable.

Sadly, many consumers who would have been better off remaining in their managed care plans discovered that insurers (and their employers) were starting to raise the premiums of those plans to unaffordable levels or dropping the plans altogether. Consumer-driven plans had become the only option for a growing number of Americans—regardless of their age, health status, or income bracket—by the time health care reform was enacted in March 2010.

FOLLOW YOUR INSURER'S LEAD

To set an example for their corporate customers, a few years ago a number of the big insurers began forcing all of their own employees into high-deductible plans. CIGNA and UnitedHealth Group were among the first to eliminate all other options for their own employees, thus encouraging their corporate customers to do the same—which insurers call "going full replacement." The new reform law will not stop employers from doing this.

Many health care experts anticipated that this would happen and warned about the likely adverse consequences of consumerism on our society. John Garamendi told reporters in 2005, while serving as California's insurance commissioner, that consumer-driven coverage would eventually result in a "death spiral" for managed care plans. This would happen, he predicted, as consumer-driven plans cherry-picked the youngest, healthiest, and richest customers while forcing managed care plans to charge more to cover the sickest patients. Garamendi's crystal ball, sadly, was clear.

While consumer-driven plans have always featured higher deductibles than traditional managed care plans, insurers initially kept the deductibles at levels ranging from one thousand to three thousand dollars. Once they had attracted or forced millions of people into these plans, however, they began moving aggressively to increase the deductibles—and in many cases raised them to levels far beyond the annual incomes of many workers. While doing this, insurers created the illusion that they were keeping the cost of coverage affordable— but in reality, they were playing a shell game.

My son, Alex, was one of thousands of other southeastern Pennsylvania residents who fell victim to this game. When Alex's policy came up for renewal at the end of 2009, he was notified by his insurer, Independence Blue Cross, that his monthly premium would increase by just $2.54—but, as is so often true with insurers, the devil was in the details. Alex's premium would increase by just $2.54, all right, but only if he switched out of his plan with a $500 deductible—which, by the way, was being discontinued—and into the company's new Personal Choice Value HSA with a $5,000 deductible. If he wished to stay in a "basic" plan similar to the one he had been in, his premium would increase by more than 65 percent.

In its cover letter to Alex and many of its other customers, Independence said that because both the cost and the usage of medical services had been going up, "we found it necessary to change the benefits structure of our Personal Choice plans to keep premiums as affordable as possible." The letter didn't mention the 65 percent increase—Alex had to do the math himself to figure that out—or that the increase was many times the rate of medical inflation.

What happened to Independence Blue Cross enrollees also happened to millions of Americans across the country. WellPoint, the largest U.S. health insurer, sent out similar notices to millions of its customers from California to Maine. According to a February 12, 2010, report issued by Maine's Bureau of Insurance (BOI), about 88 percent of enrollees in individual plans marketed by WellPoint's Anthem subsidiary in the state had deductibles of five thousand dollars per year or higher—with nearly 37 percent covered by policies with fifteen-thousand-dollar individual deductibles and thirty-thousand-dollar family deductibles.

Think about that and what it really means for a minute. The median household income in Maine was $46,419 in 2008, according to the U.S. Census Bureau. A family with that income would have to spend 65 percent of its total annual earnings on out-of-pocket expenses before its insurance company would pay any medical claims. And that's for a family earning more than half of the rest of the population. Thousands of families in Maine earn less than $30,000 a year. Imagine the ruinous number of medical bills one family could have before getting one penny of help from their insurance company. And those out-of-pocket expenses are over and above what a family would be paying in premiums. The average premium per person for individual coverage in Maine was $299 a month (approximately $3,600 a year) in 2008, according to the BOI report.

Even with that level of cost shifting from insurer to policyholders, Anthem requested approval from state regulators to raise premiums for individual plans an average of 18.1 percent in 2009. Maine's superintendent of insurance, Mila Kofman, considered the proposed increase excessive and approved a 10.9 percent increase instead. (Maine is one of the few states that give their insurance commissioner the right to reject or reduce an insurer's planned rate increases.) Contending that this would not guarantee the company the profit margin it wanted, Anthem sued the state. In an all-too-rare victory for policyholders, the Maine Superior Court affirmed Kofman's decision on April 21, 2010.

Unfortunately, cost shifting will continue, even with the enactment of reform. In a 2005 news release announcing the results of a survey of employers on the subject, which showed that more than three quarters of all U.S. companies planned to shift costs to their employees, Sandy Lutz, director of research for PricewaterhouseCoopers's Health Research Institute, said, "Shifting a greater share of spiraling health care costs to employees is a trend that is likely to continue." She added the caution that "if employers push too far, workers may opt out of coverage altogether."[7]

A separate study by benefits-consulting firm Hewitt Associates showed that the average employee contribution to company-provided health insurance increased by more than 143 percent between 2000 and 2005, while average out-of-pocket costs increased by 115 percent.[8]

SELLING THE ILLUSION OF COVERAGE

Yet another scheme to shift costs to consumers and away from insurers and employers is to enroll them in limited-benefit plans. The big insurers have spent millions of dollars acquiring companies that specialize in these plans, often providing such skimpy coverage that some insurance brokers refuse to sell them.

CIGNA markets a limited-benefit plan to midsized employers

with high employee turnover, such as chain restaurants, under the brand Starbridge Select. Not only are the benefits very limited, but the underwriting criteria would also appear to guarantee an impressive profit margin. Under the plan, the average age of an employer's workers cannot be higher than forty, and no more than 65 percent of employees can be female. (Insurers have long charged women more than men simply because they can have babies—and, consequently, maternity-related medical expenses—and are susceptible to breast cancer.) And get this: To qualify, employers must have a 70 percent or higher annual employee-turnover rate—which means that most employees won't stay on the job long enough to use their benefits. Employees also get no coverage for care related to any preexisting conditions they might need during their first six months of enrollment. Plus employees have to pay the entire premium—employers are not allowed to provide any subsidies. While a relatively small number of employers meet all these criteria, there are enough to make it very worthwhile to market the Starbridge Select plan.

There are so many restrictions built into limited-benefit contracts that there is always reduced risk to insurers, who appear only too happy to sell these policies to people who don't realize they could be ill served. Insurance companies are selling the often inadequate policies, which in some cases amount to no more than fake insurance, to keep from losing these people's business altogether. An indication of just how lucrative limited-benefit plans are is that Aetna and CIGNA were two of the biggest sponsors of the first Limited Medical & Voluntary Benefits Conference, held in October 2009 in Los Angeles.

Limited-benefit plans, coupled with high deductibles, represent the ultimate in cost shifting and are among the fastest-growing health insurance products. They're the future that insurers had in mind as they fought bitterly against reform that could jeopardize their profits. The reform bill will put a cap on the amount that an individual or family will have to pay in out-of-pocket expenses, but it will not be low enough to keep many people from having to file for bankruptcy and losing their home if they get seriously sick or injured.

KEEP SHAREHOLDERS HAPPY—AND RICH

By jacking up premiums and shifting more and more cost to their policyholders, insurers are able to manipulate an obscure ratio that is especially important to their shareholders: the medical-loss ratio (MLR). It is telling that insurers consider the amount of money paid out in medical claims to be a loss. (Some companies now call it by other names, such as the "benefit ratio," which may sound more palatable.) When an insurer lowers its MLR, it is spending less on medical care and more on overhead.

Most for-profit companies provide quarterly accountings to their investors of how well they have performed financially during the preceding three months. Shareholders of health insurance companies look for changes in two measures: earnings per share, a standard measure of profitability at all publicly traded companies, and the MLR, unique to health insurers and always reported as a percentage. An MLR of 90 percent, for example, means the insurer spent 90 cents of every premium dollar on medical care.

If an insurer reports that its MLR was lower during the preceding quarter than during the same quarter a year earlier, it means the company spent less on medical care—and therefore had more money left over to cover sales, marketing, underwriting, other administrative expenses, and, most important, profits. Such a report is considered very good news by investors and analysts—who want the MLR to decline every quarter. This, in turn, pressures insurers to be vigilant in finding ways to cut their spending on medical care, and this vigilance has paid off: Since 1993, the average MLR in America has dropped from 95 percent to around 80 percent.

One of my responsibilities at CIGNA was to handle the communication of these financial updates to the media, so I knew just how important it was for insurers not to disappoint investors with a rising MLR. Even very profitable insurers can see sharp declines in their stock prices after admitting that they have failed to trim medical expenses as much as investors expected. Aetna's stock price once fell more than 20 percent in a single day after executives disclosed that the company had spent slightly more on medical claims during the most recent quarter than in a previous period. The "sell alarm" was sounded when the company's first-quarter MLR increased to 79.4 percent from 77.9 percent the previous year.

I could always tell how busy my day was going to be when CIGNA announced earnings by looking at the MLR numbers. If shareholders were disappointed, the stock price would almost certainly drop, and my phone would ring constantly with financial reporters wanting to know what went wrong.

HOW INSURANCE COMPANY EXECUTIVES BENEFIT FROM LOWER MLRS

If anyone hates to see the MLR going up more than investors do, it is the insurance company executives and their favored senior managers—who get much of their bonus compensation in the form of stock options. When an increase in the MLR prompts investors to unload shares, the stock price will go down—and along with it, the value of an executive's stock options. The CEO and other top executives can make or lose millions in one day, depending on which way the MLR goes.

I never got close to the same pay grade as the CEO, but I nevertheless hated to see the value of my stock options go down. So, I paid close attention to the stock price for personal reasons, just as every other executive in a for-profit health insurance company does—including the medical directors who call the shots on whether to pay for expensive treatments and procedures like transplants. They know that they play a key role in reducing medical expenses, and they also stand to benefit financially if the company meets Wall Street's expectations.

Rescinding individual policies, purging small-business customers, denying claims, cheating doctors, pushing new mothers and breast cancer patients out of the hospital prematurely, and shifting costs to consumers are the ways insurance companies cut their medical expenses and keep their MLRs from inching up a decimal point or two.

While I was at the RAM expedition in Wise County, I talked to people who told me that they had health insurance, but their plans had such limited benefits or high deductibles that they couldn't afford to get the care they needed. Others told me that while they had coverage for medical care, they had lost their dental and vision benefits because their employers had stopped offering them or made the benefits so expensive that they couldn't afford them. In the euphemism-laden language that insurance executives, investors, and analysts use, these unfortunate people were the victims of "benefit buy-downs."

As I listened to their stories, I realized I was witnessing the consequences of those trends in health insurance coverage. Soon after I left my job at CIGNA in 2008, I called RAM headquarters in Knoxville and asked how many people who showed up for care at the organization's U.S. expeditions had insurance. It was about 40 percent. Small wonder when you think of all the health care that a plan with a thirty-thousand-dollar deductible won't pay for.

In fact, I learned that the demand at RAM's expeditions has increased dramatically in recent years owing to the number of people now underinsured. As a result, RAM volunteers turn away more people than they treat at many expeditions. For example, at RAM's first urban expedition, held in August 2009 at the Forum in Los Angeles, care was provided to 6,334 people. Yet despite the thousands of doctors, nurses, dentists, optometrists, and other medical professionals who volunteered their time, more than 10,000 people were turned away.

In all the years that RAM has been providing free care to

thousands of Americans, founder Stan Brock said that except for an occasional matching contribution of less than one hundred dollars, the group has not received any financial support from an insurance company.

Not even, he said, from the one he used to work for, Mutual of Omaha.

CHAPTER VII

It's All About the Money

WHEN President Bill Clinton was forced to give up on comprehensive health care reform in 1994, the damage was far more extensive than anyone could have imagined—the administration's defeat emboldened health insurance companies to totally redefine the mission and methods of an industry that now strands nearly fifty million people without insurance.

As I outlined in the previous chapter, insurers knew after the Clinton disaster that the coast was clear for them to abandon nonprofit practices, long-standing commitments to public service, and traditional insurance models and turn instead to satisfying Wall Street investors' desire to make money, by limiting spending on health care.

It may seem a distant memory, but this outcome appeared unlikely in the euphoric months after Clinton defeated President George H. W. Bush in 1992. The White House and the Democrats thought they could fulfill one of Clinton's key campaign promises: extending health coverage to millions of uninsured people while protecting the benefits of those already enrolled in public and private plans. Upset about rising health insurance premiums, most Americans said they were ready for change.[1]

Clinton also seemed mindful of voters' desire to overhaul the health care system without expanding government or raising taxes.[2] In a speech to Congress in September 1993, he announced his Health Security initiative, and it was greeted with excitement in the press. Mainstream media and political figures spoke of the plan as if it were a fait accompli. The political class chattered about history in the making, the guarantee of health insurance for all—an outcome that would rank with President Lyndon Johnson's successes in the 1960s.

Polls showed widespread public anxiety about access to adequate health care. Health costs were rising at the punishing annual rate of 8.5 percent, leaving millions uninsured and saddling doctors and hospitals with a growing burden of uncompensated care.[3] On paper, conditions were favorable for passing a comprehensive program.

In January 1993, when Clinton was inaugurated, I had just been promoted to head of communications at Humana and was reporting to Wayne Smith, the company's president. Smith reported to Humana's founder and CEO, David Jones, who had relinquished day-to-day control of the company to focus on the more pressing matter of health care reform.

That year, Jones assumed the chair of a coalition called the Healthcare Leadership Council, formed in 1990 by fifty CEOs of insurance companies, hospitals, drug companies, and medical-device manufacturers to influence reform. The CEOs didn't particularly like or trust one another because they made money in often-conflicting ways—there was the "one man's profit is another man's loss" thing at play—but the single motivation they shared was their general disdain for government regulation of their businesses. The group had tried to get President George H. W. Bush to support changes the HLC wanted, thinking it would have a better chance during his administration of getting legislation enacted that would actually eliminate existing regulations the member companies didn't like. But health care was not a priority for Bush.

So when Clinton was elected, the HLC felt a sudden sense of urgency. And for the first few months, there was a kind of uneasy honeymoon, with insurance company executives and their allies saying posi-

tive things about Clinton's approach to reform—mostly because
Clinton had indicated that his legislation would be based on a concept
the industry supported: managed competition.

The term came from an industry-friendly think tank, the Jackson
Hole Group, named after the Wyoming ski resort where the group's
members met. One of them was Larry English, who headed CIGNA's
health care operations. English also headed a coalition of big insurers
called the Alliance for Managed Care, which advocated for industry-
friendly reform. The AMC called managed competition "a private-
sector approach to health system reform that uses the marketplace
and the power of informed consumer choice to achieve better coverage, while improving quality and cutting cost." Other advocates of
the concept were Alain Enthoven, then a professor of economics at
Stanford University, and Dr. Paul Ellwood, a pediatric neurologist
who had coined the term "health maintenance organization" during
the Nixon years. The big insurers loved managed competition because
it was based on the premise that government would have minimal
involvement.

During his campaign, Clinton embraced the managed competition approach, and within weeks of being inaugurated he sent Ira Magaziner (who was helping Hillary Clinton develop legislation that the
White House would eventually present to Congress) to Jackson Hole to
meet with the group.

The honeymoon ended when it became clear that the Clintons and
Magaziner were considering not only more regulation of the insurance
industry but also federally imposed spending caps—or "global budgets,"
as Democrats called them—to control rising health care costs. Insurance executives and their allies wasted no time attacking price controls. Humana's Jones called global budgets a "top-down" approach
that would amount to "rationing by chaos . . . a trap to be avoided at
all costs."

When the Clintons unveiled their plan several months later, the
insurers were already on the attack, both visibly and behind the scenes.

CIGNA executives, in a newsletter to employees and customers, lamented that the Clintons' proposed reform legislation "shed many essential free-market principles upon which managed competition functions."

The HLC office in Washington became a war room for the special interests united in their opposition to price controls. Headed by Pamela Bailey, who had been deputy director of Ronald Reagan's Office of Public Affairs, the HLC was already operating full tilt as a message-creation and -distribution factory when I attended my first meeting there during my final weeks as a Humana employee. (I was already talking to a recruiter about taking my eventual job at CIGNA's health care operations in Connecticut.)

Another former Reagan appointee, Claire del Real, headed the HLC's communications operation. Del Real had been acting assistant secretary for public affairs at the Department of Health and Human Services. Her husband, Juan del Real, had been HHS's general counsel.

It became clear to me that the HLC was going to conduct a fear-mongering campaign against the Clinton plan that the insurance companies, drug companies, and hospital systems could not conduct themselves without appearing self-serving. They needed a front group to do it for them, and the HLC fit the bill.

It didn't help Clinton that the White House plan was intimidating in scope and complexity (or that the initiative was formulated by political and academic "elites" convened behind closed doors by the president's wife). The heart of the plan was the creation of mandatory purchasing cooperatives in each state that would insert themselves into the insurance relationship of employers and patients. In addition to establishing global budgets to limit total spending on health care, the Clintons wanted to place caps on health insurance premiums and create a federal council to review prices for new drugs. They also wanted drug companies to pay rebates to the Medicare program.

The concept was without precedent, and the administration had difficulty comparing it to anything that people recognized. Haunted by the Reagan-Bush era that had just ended, Democrats were loath to own up to the reality that Health Security would be an expansion of governmental authority that would benefit the public. The administration instead tried to portray it as a huge, voluntary, nongovernmental program. But this created the opening that the health insurance industry needed to undercut Clinton without appearing to be intransigent or hostile to the interests of American families or, at least initially, even being very visible in attacking the plan.

As the *National Journal* noted in a story about the Clinton plan headlined "Lost Cause," the HLC mounted a multipronged attack including grassroots organizing, lobbying by corporate chief executives, and public relations efforts. At the same time, it ran ads around the country raising the specter of health care rationing and warning of bureaucratic interference with patients' rights.[4] All of this was done under the name of the HLC, not the individual companies that funded it.

Although it was a propaganda operation, the HLC described itself as "the exclusive forum for the nation's health care leaders to jointly develop policies, plans, and programs to achieve their vision of a 21st century system that makes affordable, high-quality care accessible to all Americans." It also bragged that "because of the broad scope of the HLC membership, HLC is well known by congressional members and staff as an integral source for comprehensive information on health care issues."

In reality, what the HLC wanted was reform that would benefit its member companies far more than "all Americans." It wanted fewer, rather than more, government regulations. One of its initial goals was to exempt employers of all sizes from state insurance mandates. Had the HLC been successful in getting that accomplished, state insurance commissioners would have virtually no authority to regulate health insurers.

An effective tool in the health insurers' kit turned out to be the Goddard Claussen–produced series of TV commercials starring "Harry and Louise," a fictional middle-aged, middle-class couple. One of the ads showed Harry and Louise sitting at the kitchen table worriedly discussing the benefits and choices they would lose under a "government-controlled" health plan. Funded by the Health Insurance Association of America, the ad campaign truly resonated—a vast majority of Americans enjoyed employer-sponsored health insurance, and they worried about what Health Security might do to their benefits. Opinion polls began showing public support slipping after the messages from Harry and Louise, the mild suburbanites, hit the airwaves.[5]

But while the "Harry and Louise" ads got much of the credit for killing the Clinton plan, the HLC's stealth campaign was arguably more effective where it counted. The HLC aired radio ads blasting Health Security and warning that it could lead to "Washington bureaucrats deciding how much care can be given to you and your family." The Ridley Group, a Washington-based communications firm, produced the ads, which encouraged listeners to call a toll-free number to tell Congress how much they hated the Clinton plan. When callers dialed the number, they reached Bonner and Associates, a "grassroots" lobbying firm that patched the calls through to members of Congress.

The HLC's Bailey told the *National Journal* that at the peak of the ad campaign, about five thousand calls a day were being generated. The campaign was targeted to specific committees and specific votes—and was revised weekly after strategy meetings at the HLC's office.

I attended many of those strategy sessions, first on behalf of Humana and then, beginning in July 1993, on behalf of CIGNA. The group's operations were comprehensive and sophisticated. Its lobbying and PR activities were focused on all of the congressional districts where voters were about evenly split between Democrats and Republicans. The insurance industry would do exactly the same thing fifteen years later during the recent health care debate.

One guiding force behind the HLC's strategic operations was Blair Childs, with whom I worked closely in 1993 and 1994. Childs, who had run a media, grassroots, and coalition-building campaign for the health-insurance-industry-funded American Tort Reform Association in the late 1980s and had also served a stint at Aetna, knew the importance of coalition building and stealth PR in achieving corporate political objectives.

During a speech in 1994 to a group of PR professionals, Childs talked openly about what he had done for health insurers.[6] "The insurance industry was real nervous," he said. "Everybody was talking about health care reform . . . We felt like we were looking down the barrel of a gun." To take control of the debate, Childs said, the industry had to form coalitions, which he explained were essential "to provide cover for your interest. We needed cover because we were going to be painted as the bad guy. You also get strength in numbers. Some have lobbying strength, some have grassroots strength and some have good spokespersons . . . Start with the natural, strongest allies, sit around a table and build up . . . to give your coalition a positive image." He added that to defeat the Clinton plan, the coalitions drew in "everybody from the homeless Vietnam veteran to some very conservative groups. It was an amazing array, and they were all doing something."[7]

It was indeed an amazing array, and I was quite proud to be a part of the effort to make sure that the Clintons' vision of reform would never be realized. At the time, I was still a true believer in both the concept of managed care and the idea that the free market could work in health care if the government would just get out of the way. It never occurred to me that fearmongering and fake grassroots initiatives were anything to get worked up about, because they were being used to defeat a reform plan that I thought would be bad for the country—and for the companies that enabled me to pay my mortgage.

By early fall of 1994, shortly after HLC's radio campaign ended, the Clinton plan was officially dead. Senate majority leader George Mitchell pulled the plug on reform on September 26 when it became clear he would never have enough votes in the Senate to overcome a filibuster. "The $300 million that the health insurance and other lobbies had spent to stop health care reform was well invested," Clinton wrote ten years later in his memoir.[8]

Republican allies of the HLC did their jobs during the debate by debunking the Democrats' narrative and claiming that the characterization of the U.S. health care system as dysfunctional was a canard. They argued that the United States actually had the world's finest health care delivery system and that Clinton's government-managed health care would place significant barriers between Americans and their doctors.

A large part of the political effort by the GOP to kill the initiative was aimed at bringing back the "glory" of the Reagan years by continuing to deregulate the economy. The stakes couldn't have been higher. Antigovernment conservatives pulled out all the stops, according to Theda Skocpol, a Harvard University sociologist, who wrote in a 1995 postmortem,

> Ideologues and think tanks launched lurid attacks on the plan.
> Small-business members of the National Federation of Independent Business and other associations mobilized against [a provision in the bill that would have required all employers to offer coverage to their employees]. Portrayals of the plan as a bureaucratic takeover by welfare-state liberals were regular grist for Rush Limbaugh and other right-wing hosts of hundreds of news/talk radio programs that reach tens of millions of listeners (indeed, more than half of voters surveyed at polling places in the November 1994 election said they tuned in to such shows, and the most frequent listeners voted Republican by a 3-to-1 ratio). Similarly, Christian Coalition groups, already attacking Bill and Hillary Clinton on cultural issues, began to devote substantial resources to the anti–health care reform crusade. Moderate Republicans who had initially been inclined to work out some sort of compromise

began to backpedal in the face of such antireform pressures from within their own party. And interest groups whose leaders had been prepared to bargain over reforms soon were pressured by constituents and Republican leaders to back off from cooperation with the Clinton administration and congressional Democrats.[9]

REFORM DEFEAT LOOSENED
UNBRIDLED GREED

Without energetic support in Congress, the initiative simply ran out of political and parliamentary steam. "The president and his allies could have done a better job than they did of explaining the regulatory mechanisms in their plan," wrote Skocpol. "But even if the Clinton administration had communicated more effectively, the plan might still have gone down to a defeat that backfired badly against the Democrats. The bedrock fact is that the Clinton plan promised too much cost-cutting regulation and not enough payoffs to organized groups and middle-class citizens pleasantly ensconced in the existing U.S. health care system."[10]

That November, the political bill for Clinton's miscalculations came due. Riding a wave of antigovernment sentiment that the health care reform battle had aroused, Republicans took advantage of an anemic Democratic turnout and won control of the House for the first time in forty years and the Senate for the first time since 1986. The party coalesced around its Contract with America to restore the Reagan revolution. Republicans would shrink government, reduce taxes, reform the welfare system, impose term limits, and fulfill all the dreams conservatives held dear. The contract made no mention of health care.

Against this backdrop, the industry with the most to lose under Clinton's health care reform suddenly stood tall and unscathed. Instead of facing new regulations that threatened the health insurance business model, insurers faced conditions that were perfect for letting the invisible hand of capitalism spread aggressive management of medical care across the country—and create enormous profits in the process.

It's clear that voters were frightened away from Health Security by the specter—conjured up by the insurance industry and its business and political allies—of government bureaucrats coming between them and their doctors. What Americans got instead was private insurance companies doing exactly the same thing.

Within months, the Blue Cross and Blue Shield Association took a little-noticed but monumental step. The trade group, a bastion of nonprofit health insurers that included the founders of the modern health insurance system, amended its bylaws to permit members to convert into public-stock companies.[11] In one fell swoop, the association's new rules delivered a for-profit jolt to the health insurance industry. The change refocused health plans away from local service and nonprofit status. They now dreamed of consolidation into for-profit, national entities that could crush weaker local competitors.

For years, the Blues had enjoyed state and federal tax breaks granted by state lawmakers who recognized their special status as "insurers of last resort." But after Medicare and Medicaid were created in 1965, the Blues no longer had to cover millions of elderly, disabled, and poor Americans—fundamentally changing the private health insurance market.

The Blues defended their transformation as necessary for raising money from investors to keep pace with commercial competitors unburdened by public service traditions. They also avoided discussing increasingly sophisticated "underwriting" techniques designed to help avoid covering people with health risks—even though they were the very people who needed insurance protection. In this new environment, Blues executives claimed that consolidation would create economies of scale, spreading fixed overhead costs over larger numbers of customers and saving money for everyone.[12]

But these executives had a far simpler motivation for such mergers: They would earn bigger pay packages for managing larger businesses, and if they could convert them to for-profit companies, they stood to earn even more.

Fourteen Blue Cross plans, most of which dominated their state-wide markets, converted from nonprofits into for-profits, and by 2004 all fourteen wound up as wholly owned subsidiaries of WellPoint: the Blue Cross plans in California, most of southeastern New York, Georgia, Indiana, Missouri, Virginia, Colorado, Wisconsin, Connecticut, Maine, Kentucky, Ohio, New Hampshire, and Nevada. About one third of nearly one hundred million Blue subscribers in the United States now belong to a for-profit plan operated by WellPoint, which today has the biggest enrollment of any private insurer.

Not all the conversions went the way the Blues wanted. A few state insurance commissioners pushed back. In 2002, Kansas insurance commissioner Kathleen Sebelius, now President Obama's secretary of health and human services, rejected Blue Cross Blue Shield of Kansas's request to switch from a mutual insurance company to a stock company so it could be acquired by WellPoint. Sebelius argued that the transaction would push premiums higher after the health plan raised its profit margins to match those of other commercial insurers. The decision was politically popular, leading her to the governor's mansion in Topeka.[13]

In the same year, Maryland insurance commissioner Steven Larsen, who later joined Sebelius's team soon after Obama signed the 2010 health care reform bill, was asked by nonprofit CareFirst Blue Cross Blue Shield to allow the company to convert to for-profit status, a decision that would also affect sister companies providing Blue Cross coverage in Delaware, the District of Columbia, and northern Virginia. CareFirst's top executives claimed to be motivated by concern for the long-term welfare of the company and the millions of customers who depended on it for their well-being. The truth was that the transaction was engineered to maximize the executives' personal compensation, as revealed by an article in the *Washington Post* on September 16, 2002: "The 10 top executives of the region's largest health insurer stand to collect $47.9 million in severance benefits if state regulators allow the nonprofit CareFirst BlueCross BlueShield to be acquired by for-profit WellPoint Health Networks Inc.," it stated. "Severance packages, including payroll and excise taxes, would cost $78 million if all 10 left after a merger."

Six months later, Larsen, who is now deputy director of the U.S. Office of Consumer Information and Insurance Oversight, concluded that CareFirst's board was trying to sell the company at a below-market price and that it had failed to show that conversion was necessary for it to stay in business.[14] Time has borne out Larsen's judgment.

The consumer victories in Kansas and Maryland effectively halted Blue Cross conversions, but they did not stop nonprofit or mutual Blue Cross franchises from paying eye-popping compensation. For example, Blue Cross Blue Shield of Wyoming had only one hundred thousand members in 2007, but CEO Timothy Crilly collected a salary of $471,000, or $4.71 per member, the highest per capita rate in the nation.[15]

MONEY FOR INVESTORS, BUT NOT THE SICK AND DYING

Of course, the Blues didn't corner the market on health insurance industry consolidation. Mergers and acquisitions became routine for commercial insurers as well, and the government did nothing to limit them. All told, health insurers have been involved in more than four hundred corporate mergers since 1996, according to antitrust lawyer David Balto, a former Federal Trade Commission policy chief.[16]

As mergers and acquisitions swept the health insurance marketplace and competition waned, the Department of Justice antitrust division and the FTC stood by silently. During the Bush administration, the FTC and the DOJ took no consumer-protection anticompetitive-practices actions. The FTC's health care industries antitrust enforcement was targeted almost exclusively at providers—usually small groups of doctors, many of them in rural areas.

The result of this laissez-faire regulation was that a cartel of huge for-profit insurance companies set the tone for the entire industry. It's no coincidence that huge institutional investors, like Dodge & Cox, Barclays Bank, BlackRock, and T. Rowe Price, along with moneymen like Warren Buffett, had substantial holdings in the health insurance industry (although Buffett, significantly, sold the millions of shares he held in WellPoint and UnitedHealth Group in early 2010).

In February 2010, the AMA issued its annual report on the state of competition in the health insurance industry, and the results were alarming. In twenty-four of forty-three states covered by the AMA report, the two largest insurers had a combined market share of 70 percent or more. That was up from eighteen of forty-two states the year before. Among the 313 metropolitan markets, an astonishing 99 percent were "highly concentrated" under Department of Justice guidelines, up from 94 percent the year before. In 54 percent of metropolitan markets, at least one insurer had a market share of 50 percent or greater, up from 40 percent of metropolitan markets in 2009.[17]

"The near total collapse of competitive and dynamic health insurance markets has not helped patients," said AMA president Dr. J. James Rohack. "An absence of competition in health insurance markets is clearly not in the best economic interest of patients." The AMA urged the DOJ and state agencies to more aggressively enforce antitrust laws "that prohibit harmful mergers."

Health insurance companies have used their enormous size to engage in anticompetitive behavior, rig the system to impose unaffordable premium increases, and deliver massive and growing profits for themselves and their shareholders. As premiums have skyrocketed, insurers have cut benefits, increased out-of-pocket costs for workers, and shed millions of enrollees who can't afford insurance. Americans have been left to pay more while getting less and less. For those without enough money for private insurance and not eligible for government-sponsored coverage, there are now only two options: buy coverage that burdens them with soaring out-of-pocket costs or go "naked."

The health care marketplace has been distorted by insurance companies wielding concentrated power because of their unique role as both sellers of insurance and buyers of health care services. Insurers have run roughshod over weaker health care providers, paying independent doctors and hospitals cut-rate fees. With only a handful of large insurers operating in most local markets, weak doctors and hospitals have had no choice but to accept the offered fees, even if it's unprofitable to do so. In self-defense, many hospitals have merged or formed alliances, and many doctors have joined large group practices to have more clout at the bargaining table, contributing to an endless upward spiral in health care costs.

In markets where there still is significant competition among insurers, some of them have been able to make sweetheart deals with special providers—a region's biggest hospital, a famous academic medical center, or a children's hospital with no nearby competitor—who have used their size and stature to negotiate more favorable rates than those of other nearby providers.[18] Insurers aren't hurt by these various levels of deal making. As long as they can continue to pass costs on to consumers through higher premiums and cost sharing, insurers can't lose. In this environment, they could only be affected if competitors were to purchase the same medical services for less and use the savings to steal customers. With little competition and unfettered capacity to pass on costs, insurers have had no real need to curb growth in provider fees. Without additional choices in the marketplace, consumers have had no choice either.

Insurers have been exposed several times for rigging the system to extract as much money as possible from ratepayers while pursuing disparate negotiating tactics against providers. An investigation by the *Boston Globe* in December 2008 revealed a "gentleman's agreement that accelerated [the] health cost crisis." The chiefs of the largest provider group in Massachusetts and the state's largest health insurer made a handshake deal to avoid creating written evidence of the arrangement. In it, Blue Cross Blue Shield of Massachusetts promised to increase payments if the provider group, Partners HealthCare, ensured that no other health plan would be charged lower rates than Blue Cross.[19]

And as I've mentioned previously, insurers retain enough of your premiums to cover profits and ever-increasing executive compensation. The companies reward CEOs lavishly for raising the stock prices of their shares. In 2007, the CEOs at the ten largest publicly traded health insurance companies collected a combined total compensation of $118.6 million—an average of $11.9 million each.[20]

If it weren't for a 2006 newspaper exposé that sparked federal probes and civil lawsuits, the former CEO of UnitedHealth, William McGuire, might have gotten away with hundreds of millions of dollars in questionable compensation. The exposé found that some CEOs and board members of public companies had abused their powers by selectively choosing dates in the past for purposes of determining the value of stock options granted to their top people. Evidence showed that United backdated stock options over twelve years for McGuire, the worst example of backdating in the country, according to the *Wall Street Journal*.

McGuire ultimately agreed to give back $620 million in stock option gains and retirement pay to settle shareholder and federal government claims. Even so, he still collected $530 million in non-stock compensation while at the helm of UnitedHealth, and the settlements did not claw back stock options worth more than $800 million, according to the *WSJ*.[21]

The compensation structures that yielded McGuire's phenomenal paydays remain at the core of what happens in for-profit health insurance companies. CEOs do whatever it takes to keep share prices up. For example, WellPoint CEO Angela Braly held about seventy-nine million dollars' worth of the company's stock during the first quarter of 2010—most of it acquired through stock options. UnitedHealth CEO Stephen Hemsley held about eighty million dollars of his company's shares, which he acquired at a fraction of their value. Aetna's Ronald Williams held more than ten million dollars in shares after selling off many more millions.[22]

These personal holdings create an incentive for companies to repurchase shares of their own stock, which pump up their share prices and earnings-per-share figures by reducing the number of shares outstanding. From 2003 through 2008, the seven largest publicly traded health insurers, which cover 112 million Americans, spent $52.4 billion buying back their own shares. Companies make repurchases with excess cash on hand (drawn from billions of dollars of premium revenue flowing through their accounts each month) or borrow the money to pay for them.

CEOs calculate that the reward for big shareholders, including themselves, will often be greater if they invest available funds in more repurchases instead of improving a company's operations. When they repurchase shares, they are reducing the amount of money available to them to make the health system run more efficiently, improve the quality of care, or reduce customers' premiums.

While stock repurchasing is also common in other industries to achieve corporate goals, William Lazonick, an economist at the University of Massachusetts, says that the health insurance industry has been especially rife with share buybacks. In a February 2010 report, he wrote,

> Among the top 50 [share] repurchasers for 2000 to 2008 were the two largest corporate health insurers: UnitedHealth Group at No. 23 with $23.7 billion in buybacks, and WellPoint at No. 39, with $14.9 billion. For each of these companies, repurchases represented 104 percent of net income for 2000–2008. Over this period, repurchases by the third largest insurer, Aetna, were $9.7 billion, or 137 percent of net income, and the fifth largest, CIGNA, $9.8 billion, or 125 percent of net income. Meanwhile, the top executives of these companies typically reaped millions of dollars, and in many years tens of millions of dollars, in gains from exercising stock options. A serious attempt at health care reform would seek to eliminate the profits of these health insurers, given that these

profits are used solely to manipulate stock prices and enrich a small number of people at the top.[23]

From 2000 to 2008, the ten largest for-profit health insurers paid their CEOs a total of $690.7 million, according to corporate filings with the Securities and Exchange Commission. As outsized as the CEO pay is, it doesn't capture the full extent of the health insurance industry's wasteful overhead. In 2009, WellPoint employed thirty-nine executives who each collected total compensation exceeding $1 million, according to company documents gathered by the House Energy and Commerce Committee. And WellPoint spent more than $27 million on retreats for its staff at resorts in such destinations as Hawaii and Arizona in 2007 and 2008, the documents showed.

Compare this lavish executive compensation to that of the administrator of the Center for Medicare and Medicaid Services, who manages the health care of forty-four million elderly and disabled Americans on Medicare and about fifty-nine million low-income and disabled recipients on Medicaid. This administrator's pay tops out at $176,000 a year.

BERNIE MADOFF SHOULD HAVE BEEN AN INSURER

The health insurance industry's uniquely American, profit-driven brand of corporate governance has armed senior executives with virtual monopoly power in many metropolitan areas and has encouraged them to pursue often breathtaking rate hikes. They have had little pushback from state regulators—most insurance commissioners lack the authority to intervene, and most state legislatures have taken a passive approach. In many states, health insurers are large employers, so they are even more politically potent—and in every state, insurers are among the biggest spenders on lobbying and campaign contributions. Not only are premium hikes tolerated, but insurance commissioners in most states have no idea what's really going on inside these companies.

Private health insurers abhor transparency and public accountability regarding claim denials, underwriting rules, payments to doctors and hospitals, death rates, racial or ethnic disparities in health status, or the health outcomes of their members. They are usually allowed to protect this important information as "trade secrets."

The best example of the industry's secrecy is the medical-loss ratio, which, as I mentioned previously, is the measurement of the share of premium revenue spent on actual health care. The trend since Clinton's plan failed has been unmistakable. In 1993, the leading insurers used about 95 percent of premium dollars on medical benefits, according to the consulting firm PricewaterhouseCoopers. The merger wave and the new philosophy about health insurance pushed MLRs down sharply, so that by 2007 the number was 81 percent.

By contrast, Medicare has consistently had a ratio greater than 97 percent since 1993.[24]

Although Wall Street constantly pressures companies to reduce their MLRs, this imperative for the first time will collide with national standards, as established by the new health care reform law. Insurers are mandated now to spend at least 80 percent of premiums on medical care for the individual and small-group market (one hundred enrollees or fewer) and at least 85 percent for the large-group market.

One might think that these new requirements will benefit health care providers and patients, but you can count on insurers to game the system. They've already tried. Within days of President Obama's signing the law, WellPoint told Wall Street analysts that it had decided to "reclassify" certain categories of costs that it had previously counted as administrative expenses and move them to the medical-spending side of the equation, effectively raising its ratios without making any actual changes in behavior.

When low MLRs were needed to impress Wall Street investors,

insurance companies excluded the cost of nurse hotlines, medical reviews, and disease-management programs from medical costs. Now that the government is demanding minimum MLRs, the insurers want regulators to consider those expenses as medical costs, a clear-cut signal to investors that they will resist efforts to get them to trim profit margins. This demonstrates how important it will be for regulators to push back against the industry's reclassification attempts and other tricks and to consider the needs of consumers more than the profit-motivated wants of insurers.

WE'RE VICTIMS, NOT VILLAINS

As they initiated their rate hikes after the Clinton debacle, insurers professed to be the "victims" of rising health costs, and they have rejected any responsibility for America's health care affordability crisis. But the size of premium increases has had no relationship to real health costs—or anything else except internal greed.

From 2000 to 2008, insurers hiked premiums in employer-sponsored group health plans by 97 percent for families and 90 percent for individuals, according to the Kaiser Family Foundation. At the same time, private-insurance payments to health care providers grew by 72 percent, medical inflation increased only 39 percent, wages only 29 percent, and overall inflation 21 percent, according to government data.[25]

If the industry had chosen to raise premiums at the exact pace that it increased spending on health care from 2000 to 2008, insurers would still have made substantial profits without pushing millions of people to go without health benefits. But during those years, insurers raised family premiums 2.5 times faster than the rate of medical inflation, 3.3 times faster than that of wages, and 4.6 times faster than that of general inflation.[26]

This data refutes industry claims that insurers are best situated to manage care and costs efficiently—claims that, as an industry spokesman, I tried, with considerable success, to spin as indisputable truth. The reality, however, which became increasingly evident to me as I rose up through the ranks, is that Wall Street–driven financial imperatives trump the needs of millions of Americans.

The lack of affordable, quality coverage has meant that many Americans with medical needs are driven to financial ruin. Medical debt was a key reason for 62 percent of personal bankruptcy filings in 2007. In 2008, there were 1.07 million household bankruptcies. And as I noted previously, the lack of coverage will contribute to the deaths of about 45,000 people this year, or 123 people every day, according to Harvard Medical School researchers.

Yet in 2009, the five largest for-profit insurance companies waltzed through the worst economic downturn since the Great Depression to set records for combined profits. WellPoint, UnitedHealth Group, Aetna, CIGNA, and Humana reported total profits of $12.2 billion in 2009, up 56 percent from the previous year. It was the best year ever for big insurance.

How did they do it? Not by insuring more people. In 2009, the five companies covered 2.7 million fewer Americans in private health plans than in 2008.[27]

Throughout the health care reform debate of 2009 and 2010, top health insurance executives argued that total industry profits equal only one penny of every dollar spent in the U.S. health care system. That was a big part of the industry's effort to make people think— erroneously—that insurers have little to do with rising health care premiums. But even using their one-penny formula, that would mean the health insurance industry collected $25 billion in profits in 2009 alone. At that rate, over a ten-year period that penny of profit could finance more than 25 percent of the $940 billion health care reform law.

Health insurance company executives—including me when I was spinning for the industry—have consistently asserted that premium hikes of as high as 40 percent are necessary to cope with rising medical costs. They also like to complain that hospitals charge private insurers more to make up for lower Medicare rates. This all fits the industry's self-portrait of powerlessness in controlling medical costs—despite the fact that, collectively, the large insurers have as much purchasing clout as Medicare. WellPoint alone—with 33.6 million members as of December 31, 2009—has nearly as much purchasing power as Medicare.

A 2008 actuarial analysis commissioned by AHIP as part of the industry's propaganda campaign argued that Medicare doesn't pay hospitals enough, causing private insurers to pay well above hospitals' costs to keep them solvent. Insurance companies invoke this myth frequently in their attempts to justify soaring premiums. The nonpartisan Medicare Payment Advisory Commission (MedPAC), an independent expert panel created by Congress, refuted this argument and found that a hospital's relative market strength—not what Medicare pays—determines what a hospital is paid by private insurers.

The history of private insurers and hospital price negotiations is telling, as MedPAC explained in its March 2009 report to Congress. From 1987 through 1992, hospital profits from private payers grew, and from 1987 through 1993 the rate of hospital cost growth was above the rate of inflation for goods and services purchased by hospitals. From 1994 through 2000, insurers restrained private-payer payment rates, and hospital cost growth fell below the rate of inflation for hospital-purchased goods and services.

"By 2000, hospitals had regained the upper hand in price negotiations due to hospital consolidations and consumer backlash against managed care," MedPAC reported. With the loss in leverage over many hospitals, private insurers in turn passed along these costs through higher premiums, higher deductibles, and benefit buy-downs, the industry's euphemism for reducing benefits. "While insurers appear to be unable or unwilling to 'push back' and restrain payments to providers, they have been able to pass costs on to the purchasers of insurance and maintain their profit margins," MedPAC said.[28]

The United States has entrusted one of the most important societal functions, providing health care, to private health insurance companies that have consolidated into huge players with weak competition. More than one out of three Americans is now enrolled in a plan administered by one of the seven largest insurance companies—all of them listed on the New York Stock Exchange and owned primarily by big institutional investors.

Despite the recent reform, most analysts expect consolidation to continue as the big insurers buy smaller competitors or push them out of business. Consolidation is inevitable because the government's failure to control it has resulted in a cartel of huge insurers so influential that smaller companies will eventually have to sell out or shut down.

The industry itself is even suggesting that the law will lead to further consolidation. In the May 16, 2010, edition of the *New York Times*, WellPoint's chief financial officer said that he believed the new law would create opportunities for WellPoint to buy many of the smaller nonprofit Blue Cross plans that were still operating in the United States, because those small plans might have difficulty competing against much larger companies like his. "We have a unique opportunity to be a Blues consolidator," he said.[29]

It will not be the new law that creates opportunities for WellPoint and other big companies; it will be the fact that the government failed the public by allowing the cartel to be formed in the first place.

In the future, it will not be "Obamacare" that takes choice away from Americans, as the insurance industry and its allies contended during the recent debate. It will be the unfettered invisible hand of the marketplace.

CHAPTER VIII

An End Too Soon

WHEN she was a little girl, Nataline Sarkisyan loved to dance and sing and write poetry. She was a Girl Scout. She dreamed of growing up to be a fashion designer. She was also proud to be an Armenian American and the daughter of Grigor and Hilda Sarkisyan, who had immigrated here from Armenian communities in Lebanon and Syria when they were children.

The Sarkisyans sent Nataline to a private Armenian elementary school near their home in Los Angeles because they wanted to make sure their only daughter could speak their native language. And Nataline was so proud of her heritage that she spent part of every weekend at the Armenian Youth Federation teaching the language to other kids whose parents couldn't afford to send them to her school.

Nataline was also very religious. She loved Bible school and was always praying for her family and her friends. Her mother said they used to pray together every night. "Just the two of us. We never missed a night."

The first time I heard about Nataline was late on the Friday afternoon of December 14, 2007. I'd been traveling that day and hadn't had a chance to check my voice mail messages. There were lots, as usual, and most of them were routine—except for one from a TV station in Los Angeles that stood out because it just didn't make sense.

The reporter said she'd been told that CIGNA was refusing to cover a liver transplant for a Los Angeles teenager because her family owned a second home. I replayed the message to be sure I'd heard it correctly. I couldn't imagine why anyone at CIGNA would care if a family had a second home and, even if they did, how it would have any bearing on whether or not to cover a transplant. Nevertheless, for the sole reason that a TV reporter had called about a CIGNA health-plan member, I gave the Nataline Sarkisyan case "high profile" status.

My staff and I took every call from reporters seriously, but we gave special attention to reporters working on "horror stories," as I mentioned earlier. Typically, whenever any of us got such a call, we would arrange a conference call with senior managers, often including the chief medical officer, and sometimes even the CEO. This one didn't seem to warrant such a call—at least not yet—but I telephoned my office to find out if any other reporters had called about it.

None had, but the same TV reporter had phoned again. I asked a colleague to call her back to try to get more information and, if necessary, to e-mail her a bland statement of some kind.

E-mail had become the most common way we communicated with reporters. It enabled us to click "send" and dispatch a statement that usually had been blessed (if not already written) by an ad hoc committee of lawyers, corporate doctors, and businesspeople. With e-mail, we were sending not just a statement but a broader message: "Here's our response to your question. Take it or leave it. It's all we're going to say." More often than not, reporters would take it and not bother us for more information. They were often on a deadline, and even if they weren't, they knew from experience that they weren't going to get much more out of us.

The statement we sent to the Los Angeles TV reporter didn't acknowledge that Nataline was a CIGNA member, much less answer any specific questions about the alleged denial: "Due to federal privacy laws we are unable to confirm that this individual is a CIGNA member at this time. Cases such as this are not decided based on cost, but rather on the medical appropriateness of treatment. There is an appeals process in place whereby physicians who are not with CIGNA review a case and provide another viewpoint on the appropriateness of treatment. We always encourage our members and their physicians to make an appeal in situations where they disagree with a decision."

We hoped that would be enough to kill the story, but it wasn't. On Saturday evening, December 15, KTLA-TV aired a brief report about the case. "Members of a local family say they're living a nightmare, and they blame their insurance company," said the station's anchor, introducing the first of what ultimately would be thousands of stories about CIGNA's refusal to pay for Nataline's liver transplant.

For the first time, I started paying close personal attention to the case. Not only did I not want CIGNA to get any more bad publicity, but I also couldn't help thinking about the family. As the father of a daughter just three years older than Nataline, I couldn't help putting myself in their shoes, wondering what life would be like for my wife and me if we were fighting with an insurance company to get it to cover a lifesaving transplant for our daughter, Emily. Just thinking about it caused me to ache. I tried to quickly put it out of my mind.

Nataline had been diagnosed with leukemia on May 28, 2004, just weeks before her fourteenth birthday. After a series of chemotherapy treatments, the leukemia was in remission. "She only had two treatments left by the time of her sweet-sixteen birthday party," her mother said. A year later, though, just as she was getting ready to go to the hospital for routine blood work, she told Hilda, "I feel weird, Mom, like something is wrong with me." Something was: Her leukemia had come back.

This time, her doctors said, chemotherapy wouldn't be enough. She needed a bone marrow transplant, and it turned out that her older brother, Bedig, was a perfect match. He gladly agreed to be the donor, and CIGNA agreed to pay for it, as long as the procedure was done at a hospital in CIGNA's network, Mattel Children's Hospital at UCLA.

"We rushed to get Nataline admitted because timing is so

important," Hilda said. Nataline had to have the bone marrow transplant within a few days of a heavy dose of chemotherapy.

Although Nataline knew her leukemia was back, "you would never have thought she was even a little sick," her mother said. "She walked into the hospital smiling, knowing she would go back home soon. She looked like she was in perfect health."

IT WAS THE BEGINNING . . . OF THE END

Nataline was admitted on Monday, November 12, 2007. Across the country in Philadelphia, I, too, was having a busy, stressful Monday, starting with an eight A.M. Public Policy Council meeting at which CIGNA's lobbyists in Washington briefed my boss (general counsel Carol Ann Petren) and me on the latest talk on Capitol Hill and in the presidential campaigns about health care reform. Immediately after that, I met with one of the company's securities lawyers about a Securities and Exchange Commission filing. At one P.M., I was off to the boardroom on the seventeenth floor for an important briefing on CIGNA's Investor Day, which would be held the following Friday at the Mandarin Oriental Hotel in New York. Because the company expected Investor Day to go well—we had told investors and analysts a few days earlier that we expected the company to earn more than a billion dollars by the end of the year—I was asked if I could get a reporter from the *Wall Street Journal* to cover it.

Nataline's bone marrow transplant, eventually performed the day after Thanksgiving, went well, but serious complications soon developed, especially in Nataline's liver, stemming from the heavy chemotherapy infusion and accompanying radiation and the transplant itself. A week after the procedure, her doctors said she had to have a liver transplant.

In early December, not long after CIGNA's Investor Day, which had cost $250,000 (just feeding the 150 investors, analysts, and CIGNA executives at the six-hour meeting had cost $60,000), Nataline was taken to the ICU, where she would wait for her new liver. Knowing that insurers normally require prior authorization—a liver transplant costs about $250,000, or the same amount CIGNA had just spent in New York—her doctors contacted CIGNA's transplant unit and asked for approval.

It never occurred to the Sarkisyans that there would be problems. The biggest worry they had was whether a liver would become available and be a match for Nataline. Early in the morning a few days later, Hilda got the call she had been praying for. "Put on your best outfit, because we have the perfect fit for your daughter," she recalls one of the doctors telling her.

Because it was the Christmas season, Nataline's favorite holiday, Hilda decided on a red outfit and rushed to the hospital, grateful that Nataline would soon be getting the liver to save her life. She was stunned when one of her daughter's doctors pulled her aside and told her, "Hilda, we have a liver, but we don't have clearance from CIGNA."

"What are you talking about?" she asked him, not understanding why CIGNA would have a say in the matter. "We have insurance, and I know it covers transplants, so what kind of clearance do you need?"

Nataline was covered under a policy that her father had obtained through Mercedes-Benz, where he worked as a technician. CIGNA administered the health care benefits for the company's employees and their dependents. It was a self-insured account—Mercedes-Benz, rather than CIGNA, assumed the risk—a fact that had seemed of little consequence at the time but that the Sarkisyans would soon learn was of enormous consequence.

Nataline's doctors told the Sarkisyans that before they could get approval to proceed with the transplant, they would have to do a biopsy of Nataline's liver to satisfy a request received from a CIGNA medical director. The Sarkisyans felt they had no choice but to agree to it. "They had to cut her and get a piece of her liver just to prove to CIGNA that she needed a transplant," Hilda said.

By the time this procedure was done, however, the liver that had been a perfect match had had to be given to another patient. The family now could only wait—and pray—for another one.

Another liver did become available a few days later, but the Sarkisyans were in for yet another shock: CIGNA refused to pay for the liver transplant, even though her doctors said it was her only hope for survival—and even though the procedure CIGNA had demanded had proved that her liver was indeed failing. A CIGNA medical director sent a message to Nataline's doctors at UCLA, where hundreds of transplants are performed every year, saying that the transplant for Nataline, in his view, would be "experimental."

It had never occurred to the Sarkisyans that their daughter's fate would be in the hands of someone whom they had never met and who had never laid eyes on their daughter, much less personally examined her or assessed her condition.

When Nataline's treating physician, a professor of pediatrics in the Division of Gastroenterology, Hepatology and Nutrition at UCLA, submitted his original request for prior authorization, a CIGNA transplant case manager in Pittsburgh began the process of reviewing Nataline's medical records and the Sarkisyans' benefit plan. Three days later, she recommended that CIGNA cover the transplant. However, because Nataline by then had developed a lung infection while in the hospital and was very weak, the case manager asked the medical director of CIGNA's transplant unit to look at the case.

The medical director denied the request from Nataline's doctors, noting that the Mercedes-Benz benefit plan did not cover "experimental, investigational and unproven services." In his opinion, a liver transplant for someone in Nataline's rapidly declining state of health would fall into that category.

Within hours of receiving this denial, Nataline's treating physician and three of his colleagues at UCLA pleaded for him to reconsider, insisting that the requested transplant would not be experimental. They contended that similar patients had been shown to have a sixty-month survival rate of approximately 65 percent.

Despite the doctors' plea, CIGNA was not persuaded that there was enough documented evidence that a liver transplant for someone in Nataline's condition would be appropriate. The company stood by its decision. In communicating that it was upholding the denial, CIGNA said that the lung infection and other problems that had developed since Nataline had been admitted to the hospital would be unlikely to result in a successful outcome for Nataline and that, consequently, the surgery would not meet CIGNA's definition of medical necessity. Who was right? The reality is that in many cases, no one ever knows. If a critically ill patient dies after an insurance company refuses to pay for a doctor-ordered procedure, which often happens, it can never be proved that the patient would have even survived the procedure.

THE FAMILY FIGHTS BACK

The Sarkisyans were devastated when they got the news that CIGNA wouldn't cover the transplant—but they were not about to give up hope, Hilda in particular. She believed that she and her friends in the Armenian community might be able to mount a campaign to shame CIGNA into approving the transplant. So she immediately began contacting family and friends in the close-knit community in Los Angeles and asking them to do anything they could to draw public attention to Nataline's plight.

Nataline's godfather started making calls to reporters and TV news producers throughout L.A. and the San Fernando Valley, where the Sarkisyans live. The TV reporter who left that first voice mail message for me had just talked to him. (The information that the Sarkisyans owned a second home—actually a rental property—apparently came from a hospital employee who noticed that Nataline's mother had listed it among the family's assets on a form the hospital had asked her to fill out when Nataline had been admitted. Whether CIGNA had access to that information is unclear, but the company denied that the family's rental property was a factor in its decision.)

Nataline's story likely would have stayed local had it not been for the California Nurses Association, a politically active and media-savvy union that represents thousands of nurses throughout the state. A co-worker of Hilda's who had been a nurse contacted CNA's leadership in Oakland and asked them to get involved in the Sarkisyans' campaign. It didn't take much arm-twisting. CNA spokeswoman Liz Jacobs said the organization never considered *not* doing all it could do for Nataline.

"We've taken our oath to be patient advocates," she said, "and we will be advocates wherever the need takes us. So we were up for this."

Early on Thursday morning, December 20, CNA blanketed the media with a news release announcing a protest that would be held at eleven A.M. that day in front of CIGNA's California headquarters, in Glendale, which happens to be in the heart of the Armenian American community. The headline was sure to get the media's attention: "Life Denied: Nurses, Family of Sick Teen March on Health Insurance Company; 17-Year-Old Girl Needs Liver Transplant, CIGNA Denies."

"My daughter survived two bouts of cancer," the release quoted Hilda as saying, "and against all odds has been stable even with so many of her organs not working, only to now be told that she cannot get the only treatment that will save her life because some administrator in some office thinks it is too expensive. We needed help in standing up against this insurance provider, and of course it was the nurses who stepped forward."

My phone started ringing off the hook as soon as the nurses' release went out. I knew I had a crisis on my hands when calls poured in not only from local TV and radio stations but also from the *Los Angeles Times*, CNN, and NBC—and even from the general public. The release, which was posted on the home page of CNA's Web site, also appealed to the public to call CIGNA demanding that it "provide the care Nataline needs."

The nurses were also making a political statement with the

protest. The California legislature was embroiled in a debate on reforming the state's health care system, and CNA, which has long supported a single-payer system that would ban private insurers, cited Nataline's situation as a reason why state lawmakers should reject a reform plan supported by Governor Arnold Schwarzenegger and some legislative leaders.

"CIGNA's refusal of Nataline's liver transplant—overruling the urgent appeals of an array of doctors and nurses—is indicative of the failures of the new health care plan sponsored by Arnold Schwarzenegger and [Assembly Speaker] Fabian Núñez," the release said. "That plan, which is actively supported by CIGNA, requires every single Californian to purchase insurance products from companies like CIGNA, but does not address the problem of denial of care evident in this situation."

As soon as I heard about the news release—from a reporter who called asking for CIGNA's reaction to it—a colleague and I immediately began alerting the company's top executives. The first person I forwarded the release to, of course, was my boss, Carol Ann Petren.

When Petren responded to my e-mail by asking if I would have the draft of a policy paper on her desk first thing the next morning, I knew she hadn't grasped the significance of what was happening. I immediately ran up the stairs from my office on the sixteenth floor to hers on the seventeenth and interrupted a meeting she was in.

After I stressed what it meant that the national media was covering a protest at our headquarters in California, she realized she had better brief our CEO, Ed Hanway, whose office was on the other end of the hall from hers. She called him herself and then asked her assistant to track down two other executives: David Cordani, then president of CIGNA HealthCare, and Dr. Jeffrey Kang, the company's chief medical officer. Hanway was in Petren's office in a matter of minutes. Cordani and Kang, who worked in Bloomfield, Connecticut, where CIGNA's health care operations were based, joined us by phone.

Kang, whom CIGNA's transplant medical director had briefed a few days earlier, explained the reasoning behind the denial and said that based on what the medical director had told him about Nataline's worsening condition, he supported the decision not to cover the transplant. He added, however, that he had ordered an expedited external review of the case, and the results were expected the next day.

Waiting until the next day to hear from the reviewers was completely out of the question. TV crews were already setting up in front of CIGNA's Glendale offices, so our discussion quickly turned to the PR damage that Nataline's story would do to the company. As I always did in situations like this, I explained the PR consequences—the likely damage to the company's reputation—if we didn't relent and agree to cover the transplant. I noted that it would be different if the patient were an older person. Reporters probably would not have found the story at all compelling if the patient had been a forty-five-year-old man. The fact that the patient was a sweet-looking seventeen-year-old girl, whose smiling face had been seen by thousands of TV viewers in Southern California, made the story irresistible to the media. There was no way the company would be perceived as anything other than a cold, heartless corporation if we didn't give a teenage girl a fighting chance to live, even if the odds weren't that good that she'd survive.

Because the scheduled protest was attracting so much media attention, it was clear we would need outside public relations support to help deal with what could become the biggest PR crisis in company history. The first person Petren mentioned was Larry Rand, highly regarded in the corporate world for his crisis communications skills. Rand was one of the founders of Kekst and Company, a New York firm that specializes in investor relations and financial PR for publicly traded companies. CIGNA had Kekst on retainer so that Rand and his staff would be available whenever we needed them.

Hanway agreed that we needed them now.

Rand was in a meeting when Petren called him. His assistant said she'd have him call her back later.

"No, I need him right now," Petren told her. "It's urgent. Tell him Ed [Hanway] is here with me."

Rand was on the phone in minutes, and when Petren told him about the protest, he didn't need to hear anything else.

"Look, Carol, you have to make this go away. Approve the transplant—now."

Although I had given the same advice, Hanway and Petren needed to hear it from an outside expert. If Nataline died, CIGNA would be blamed for her death, and the resulting publicity would be so bad that the company could lose customers. I added that it would just be a matter of time before one of the presidential candidates seized on the story—possibly elevating it to a disaster for the entire industry.

The group quickly agreed that damage control was of paramount importance. Cordani, who as president of CIGNA's health care division had the most to lose, made the decision: CIGNA itself would pay for the transplant, using its own money rather than asking Mercedes-Benz to cover it. I was relieved. I was certain that even though the media would report that CIGNA had caved to pressure, the bad publicity would be over soon and people would forget the case or at least forget that CIGNA was the insurance company involved. There would be no long-term reputational damage.

I was just as relieved, though, for Nataline's family. This harrowing and frightening episode in their lives just might have a happy ending. I imagined how joyous and hopeful my wife and I would be to hear from our insurance company—which would be CIGNA—that a procedure that might save Emily's life had been given "clearance."

I sent a quick e-mail to AHIP's PR staff to let them know that CIGNA would soon notify the family that it would cover the transplant, because they, too, were being inundated with calls. Before we could say anything about it to the media, however, someone had to get word to Nataline's family and doctors. Kang said he would make sure that the transplant case manager reached out to them right away. The other thing that needed doing right away was crafting the words to explain why we had changed our minds. We'd have to explain it in a way that didn't look like we were caving in—or setting a precedent that could nip us in the future.

It was my job to figure out how to say that CIGNA was now agreeing to approve a transplant even though we still believed we'd been right to deny it in the first place—and that our change of heart had nothing to do with the bad publicity.

RIGHT DECISION, BUT A LITTLE TOO LATE

As I ran downstairs to start writing, I knew my staff would be happy to hear about the reversal. We had all gotten caught up in the story emotionally and were hoping that Nataline would be able to get the transplant and that it wouldn't be too late. Although the prevailing belief was that Nataline's chances of survival were slim—even if she got the transplant—I didn't want to believe it. I still imagined a happy outcome, with Nataline walking out of the hospital in a few weeks with her mom and dad and brother.

I also knew that no one would really believe that CIGNA had changed its mind solely out of empathy for Nataline and her family. But I was willing to spin it that way.

I was under the gun to write the statement and get it to Petren and the others for their review, but I decided to quickly check my e-mail first to see if there were any new developments or media inquiries. I couldn't believe what I saw. E-mails were literally pouring in—at least five hundred more than when I had left for Petren's office. A few were from the media, but most were from people all over the country who'd heard about CIGNA's refusal and were writing to express their anger and outrage. I read a few and then alerted security because some were wishing harm to my family and me. I had to ignore most of them, for the time being anyway, because I had to begin writing what CIGNA as a company would say to the Sarkisyans and the world. About an hour before the start of the protest in California, I finished a draft of what would be the core of both our media statement and the letter to Nataline's father.

The letter was the first priority, and after numerous edits it was ready to go. "Dear Mr. Sarkisyan," it began. "We received an appeal request on Dec. 17, 2007. We understand you are appealing the medical necessity denial for a liver transplant for your daughter, Nataline. After reviewing the information submitted with your appeal request and the terms of your benefit plan, I am pleased to let you know that on Dec. 20, 2007, CIGNA HealthCare has decided to make an exception in this rare and unusual case, and we will provide coverage should Nataline's health care providers determine to proceed with the requested liver transplant. We are making this decision on a one-time basis, based on the unusual circumstances of this matter, although the treatment, if provided, would be outside the scope of the plan's coverage and despite lack of medical evidence regarding the effectiveness of such treatment."

I also had my media statement ready to blast to the media as soon as the letter was hand delivered to the Sarkisyan home.

With just ten minutes to go before the protest was to begin, I still didn't have confirmation that the letter had been delivered, so I started calling around to find out what was going on. There was a hitch no one had anticipated: The Sarkisyans were not at home, and no one knew where to find them.

It occurred to me that they probably were on their way to the protest. So I turned on the TV in my office, and sure enough, CNN was broadcasting live from the front of CIGNA's Glendale offices, and I could see a woman in the crowd who I assumed was Nataline's mother amid what looked like scores of nurses carrying signs with Nataline's picture and the message CALL CIGNA TODAY. The crowd was chanting, "No more denials, no more denials, health care for all *now*."

I called CIGNA's top lawyer in California, Bill Jameson, and told him he would have to send someone right away to tell the Sarkisyans that CIGNA would pay for the transplant. Hilda had already been interviewed on camera and clearly didn't know.

A few minutes later, I saw someone whisper in her ear. I could tell she was getting the good news. "CIGNA just approved!" she screamed.

The campaign had worked. CIGNA had been pressured into reversing the denial. Grigor Sarkisyan gave his wife a big hug. They looked so relieved and so happy.

The crowd cheered. Tears were streaming down the faces of many of the protesters.

I was just as happy as they were—and just as relieved.

Within an hour, CNA issued a news release with the headline "CIGNA Capitulates to Patient Revolt. Following Massive Protest, Insurer Authorizes Transplant for 17-year-old Nataline Sarkisyan. CNA-Sponsored Protest Sparks Flood of Calls from Across U.S."

"CIGNA had to back down in the face of a mobilized network of patient advocates and health care activists who would not take no for an answer," the release quoted CNA executive director Rose Ann DeMoro as saying.

I would never acknowledge it publicly, but DeMoro, of course, was right. CIGNA had capitulated. My job now was to spin the reversal in a convoluted way that would make people think the media attention, the protest, the calls, and the e-mails had nothing to do with it.

"Our hearts go out to Nataline and her family as they endure this terrible ordeal," the media statement began. Then there was this fifty-nine-word whopper of a sentence that only a lawyer could love: "Based on the unique circumstances of this situation, and although it is outside the scope of the plan's coverage and despite the lack of medical evidence regarding the effectiveness of such treatment, CIGNA Health-Care has decided to make an exception in this rare and unusual case and we will provide coverage should she proceed with the requested liver transplant."

The statement ended with this: "Our thoughts and prayers are with Nataline and her family at this difficult time."

That last part was true, at least for me. My thoughts and prayers actually were with Nataline and her family, as were those of many CIGNA employees. I felt a little queasy about writing it, though, because I knew it was a PR contrivance—and one we used whenever we had to issue a statement in such circumstances. PR people know that in situations like this one, it is important to convey how sympathetic and caring we are.

I went home late, exhausted, but knowing that the stress of my day was nothing compared to what the Sarkisyans had gone through. I was happy for them and hoped they would all get much-needed rest before Nataline's transplant.

But a few minutes after ten P.M., my phone rang at home. There would be no need for CIGNA to cover the transplant after all. Nataline had just died.

A LIFE SLIPS AWAY

Hilda Sarkisyan had no idea her daughter was so close to death when talking to the reporters in front of CIGNA's offices. "I told the media my daughter was going to be fine," she said. "She'll be getting the transplant."

However, when she arrived at the hospital after the protest, many friends and family members were already there. Her husband, in fact, had slipped away from the protest and returned to the hospital alone after his sister had called to tell him that Nataline's condition had taken a turn for the worse. Hilda found out later that many of her relatives and friends had learned before she did that Nataline was not going to recover.

"I was shocked to see so many people there," she said. "Even the archbishop was there. One of the main leaders of the Armenian community came, and the next thing you know, my husband, my uncle and my aunt, everybody was staring at me. Then my husband said, 'Hilda, I love you.'

"'Why did you say that?' I thought. We're not like that. We love each other, but we don't say that in public.

"I said, 'Okaaay.'

"'Hilda,' he said, 'our daughter just passed away.'

"They had to put me in a wheelchair."

With tears streaming down her face, she searched in her purse for a notepad. "I just began to write," she said. "I had done everything I could to save Nataline, but I knew my work was not over. I felt actually that my real work was just beginning. I promised Nataline as I said good-bye to her that I was going to make sure people understood that what happened to her, what happened to our family, could happen to them, too."

THE SPIN BEGINS

When I heard that Nataline had died, I knew that my real work had just begun, too. My top priority—the first responsibility listed in my job description—was to "protect, defend and enhance" the company's reputation. The size of my raise and bonus depended on just how well I managed to do that, and I knew I would play a central role in a weeks-long, all-out damage-control campaign. I would have to convince the media and the public—in a very nuanced and subtle way—that CIGNA, despite its reversal, had been right in denying coverage for the transplant in the first place, that it had, in fact, had a responsibility to its customers to refuse to pay for it.

It turned out to be both my biggest and my last attempt to influence public opinion on behalf of an industry I had served for nearly two decades.

My heart wasn't in it. On reflection, I was actually grieving, although I didn't realize it at the time. What I did know was that I didn't feel up to the task of spinning. I felt, instead, burned out. But I had a job to do, and I had to do it. Whether I liked it or not, I was going to be the company's main voice on the case, although I would enlist our chief medical officer, Kang, to talk with the media as well. One of the things I had learned years ago was that executives with an M.D. after their names were especially influential with reporters when the stories pertained to patient care. Whenever I could manage it, I would try to get CIGNA's point of view delivered in print by a medical director, if for no other reason than to have the M.D. appear in the story—especially if it was a horror story.

The first thing I did after I learned of Nataline's death was brief my boss, Petren. The second thing I did was call the media-monitoring services I used and ask them to send me every story that appeared anywhere in the world, in any medium—print, broadcast, or online— as soon as possible. Third, I started writing the media statement we would begin using the next day.

"Our deepest sympathies are with the Sarkisyan family as they mourn the death of Nataline," I wrote. "All of us at CIGNA send our thoughts and prayers to those who were touched by Nataline's life." I knew I had to start it that way, and it was heartfelt, but it nevertheless seemed like I was writing those sentiments only because it was a PR necessity.

I went on to note, in awkward prose, that CIGNA had agreed to cover the transplant "even though there was no medical evidence regarding the effectiveness of a liver transplant in this rare case, and no coverage for this procedure under the health plan chosen by the employer who provided health benefits to the Sarkisyan family." I added that CIGNA had a responsibility to its customers "to make medically appropriate decisions based on scientific and clinical evidence."

Petren and others who reviewed the statement made edits for legal reasons that I thought made the language even more awkward, but there was nothing unusual about that. Lawyers always had the last word when litigation was possible or anticipated.

The news coverage before Nataline's death, significant as it was, paled in comparison to the avalanche of media reports and blog posts that began almost immediately after. The first batch retrieved by the monitoring services went on for pages. I only had to read the headlines to grasp how damaging the publicity was going to be.

The one bit of good news for CIGNA was that the company was not mentioned by name in most of the headlines. People had to read or listen further to know or remember that CIGNA was the company. This was not much of a silver lining, because most of the broadcast stories did include clips from the protest in front of CIGNA's Glendale building—and the company's turquoise "tree of life" logo, with the tagline "Business of Caring" below it, appeared in many of the news reports.

My staff and I were quickly overwhelmed. It was not possible for us to talk to every reporter who called seeking comment or an on-camera interview. I asked my assistant to get every reporter's e-mail address and then send them our statement with a note telling them they could attribute it to me as the company's spokesman. I returned a few calls, but only to reporters at the major newspapers and networks. We had to have help.

Petren had been impressed with the way that PR firm APCO had earlier worked behind the scenes on behalf of the industry to discredit Michael Moore's *Sicko*. After a brief conversation with Robert Schooling, the APCO executive who had led the *Sicko* work, she hired the firm. In addition to Schooling, APCO would assign Myron Marlin, senior vice president and senior strategist, to the account. A lawyer as well as a PR guy, Marlin had been director of public affairs at the Department of Justice during the Clinton administration. Schooling and Marlin would become active participants in the twice-daily "California case" strategy sessions and conference calls led by Nicole Jones, our corporate secretary.

Jones's "lead team," as she called the group, also included Hanway, Cordani, Kang, Brian Benjet (who headed litigation for CIGNA), G. William Hoagland (the company's Washington-based vice president of government affairs, who had been a top aide to Senate majority leader Bill Frist), and Larry Rand and Lissa Perlman, both of Kekst. Karen

Ignagni, president of AHIP, also called in occasionally, as did her lieutenant, Mike Tuffin, who led strategic communications for the trade group.

Benjet was a member of the lead team because the Sarkisyans had hired Mark Geragos, often referred to as the "lawyer to the stars" (Michael Jackson was among his famous clients), to represent them. Geragos had also long been active in the Armenian community in Los Angeles. Hilda Sarkisyan said that she and her husband had retained him initially in their efforts to get CIGNA to pay for the transplant; the day after Nataline died, he held a press conference to announce that he would be filing a lawsuit against CIGNA.

"My reading of the statute is clear that this corporation had the mental state that they consciously disregarded her life," Geragos said at the press conference. In addition to filing his own lawsuit, he said, he planned to ask the U.S. attorney in Los Angeles, Thomas O'Brien, to press murder or manslaughter charges against the company that "maliciously killed" Nataline because it didn't want to bear the expense of her transplant and aftercare.

After those comments made headlines, Benjet hired Debra Yang, who was O'Brien's predecessor as U.S. attorney until she resigned in 2006 to join a big international law firm. The lead team also started a "Geragos watch" to monitor his actions and comments. As part of that watch, Yang arranged to have someone attend Nataline's funeral on December 28 and report back if the company was mentioned in any way during the service.

Schooling and Marlin's responsibilities were to help create a detailed communications plan that would encompass the same tactics that APCO had used in its behind-the-scenes campaign against *Sicko*. The plan was ready for review by the lead team on December 30 and, like the *Sicko* strategy, relied heavily on the firm's ability to place stories with reporters, editors, and producers it had good relationships with and to get "third parties" to convey CIGNA's messages.

The main objective was to try to drive reporting on the case to the broader issue of tough decisions that have to be made about the allocation of scarce organs and whether someone in Nataline's condition would have been approved for a transplant in any other health care system around the world. The point was to disabuse the media, politicians, and the public of the notion that Nataline would have gotten the transplant if she had lived in Canada or France or England or any other developed country.

APCO planned an aggressive outreach to reporters and pundits likely to be most receptive to such "big picture" stories and to be sympathetic to CIGNA's point of view. APCO would also draft and work to place letters to the editor and op-ed pieces "to set the record straight" if a newspaper carried a negative story or editorial about the case. Knowing that the industry was worried that advocates of health care reform would seize on the case as a reason why the American health care system needed to be drastically overhauled, APCO would use the op-eds as vehicles to also argue that a government-run system would not keep such cases from happening in the future, and to suggest that a more useful role for government would be to develop a national policy on coverage for "experimental" treatments.

The pundits APCO proposed to reach included some of the most famous TV health care reporters and commentators, and the list of third-party advocates was a who's who of reliable insurance industry allies, including many of the same people APCO had enlisted earlier to help in its *Sicko*-bashing campaign. All were associated with conservative think tanks, big-business organizations, or legal-reform groups that the health insurance industry had reached out to many times in the past for help disseminating messages that could not be traced to AHIP or any insurer. And in anticipation that Geragos would continue generating stories about his lawsuits, APCO had a second list of pundits to argue that America was plagued with "frivolous lawsuits" that were driving up the cost of health care.

A third list was doctors whom APCO or CIGNA would ask to be third-party "experts" on organ transplants. They would be available to speak with reporters or to write op-eds, if necessary, that would convey the company's point of view.

AFTER THE TARGETS COMES THE SPIN

The APCO plan also included a list of approved talking points and a comprehensive set of potential questions and answers that all of the spokespeople would be required to study before talking with anyone in the media.

Two days before Schooling and Marlin laid out the communications plan to the lead team in Philadelphia, Nataline was laid to rest in California. Shortly before her burial, the Sarkisyan family led hundreds of mourners, many of them wearing pink (Nataline's favorite color), into St. Mary's Armenian Apostolic Church, the spiritual heart of the Los Angeles Armenian community. (Debra Yang reported to us that the people who spoke did not use the occasion to condemn CIGNA but to remember what Nataline had meant to them and to others.)

After the eulogies were delivered, Nataline was buried in a white coffin. Her heartbroken father had insisted on white. To keep her spirits up while she was in the hospital, he had promised Nataline that he would buy her a white Mustang as a graduation present. "I had to buy her a white coffin instead," he told me two years later when I met the Sarkisyans in their home.

APCO had predicted that a presidential candidate, probably John Edwards, would begin talking about the Sarkisyan case. They were right. Edwards even invited the Sarkisyan family to join a campaign stop in New Hampshire. Elizabeth Edwards, campaigning with her husband, introduced the family at an emotional town hall meeting in Manchester on January 6, 2008.

"I feel empty inside," Hilda Sarkisyan told the crowd. "But this is not only about my daughter Nataline; it's about the whole world, every one of you. This could have happened to any of us. We have to put a stop to these people. They cannot tell us who's going to live and who's going to die. Right now I am here for her. We have to make a change."

After this appearance, however, media interest in the case began to wane. Thanks to the successful implementation of the APCO strategy, many of the stories that did appear focused more on CIGNA's side of the story than on the Sarkisyans'. By this time, reporters writing about the case were looking for fresh angles, and the APCO team and I were pushing those angles to select media.

Of course, I played a key role in this effort. One of my jobs was to arrange interviews for Kang with reporters with whom I had developed good relationships and who might be more inclined to write stories from CIGNA's point of view. I scored several coups when favorable or at least balanced articles began to appear in important publications, including *Forbes* and the *Wall Street Journal.* These were especially important because they would be read by the CEOs and benefits managers of CIGNA's corporate customers, some of whom were already calling us to get statements they could use with their employees who were enrolled in CIGNA plans.

I couldn't have been happier to see the headline on the January 8 *Forbes* story: "Does CIGNA Deserve All the Blame?" Reporter David Whelan, an influential reporter whom I had allowed to interview Hanway several weeks earlier at CIGNA's Investor Day in New York, included the Kang quotes I had hoped he would use. He also left out a quote I was praying he would not use.

"CIGNA's medical director, Jeffrey Kang, a physician who used to be a high-ranking official with the Centers for Medicare and Medicaid Services, says there is no way that CIGNA can stop doctors from performing a liver transplant," Whelan wrote. "A national organization called the United Network for Organ Sharing manages the waiting lists. One of UNOS's principles is that patients should get transplants regardless of their financial means. 'Some people have said we denied a liver,' Kang says. 'But the reality is we only denied paying for it.'"

During the telephone interview (I was also on the line, as I was on all interviews with CIGNA's top executives), Whelan pressed Kang, who was in his office in Connecticut, on whether CIGNA had had any financial incentives to deny the transplant. Staying on message, Kang said that because Grigor Sarkisyan's plan was a self-insured account, it would have been the employer's money—not CIGNA's—that would have been used to pay for the transplant.

"You must have some financial incentives to keep costs down, right?" Whelan followed up. "The short answer is no," Kang replied.

Then, to my astonishment, he kept going: "I have to be honest, though. If we have a three-year contract with an employer, if that employer is looking to rebid that contract, they'll say, 'Let's look at what CIGNA's track record was overall and see what we can get from a competitor.'" In other words, Kang was acknowledging that to keep accounts like Mercedes-Benz, an insurer had to demonstrate that it did a good job of holding down medical expenses.

I breathed a sign of relief when Whelan moved on to another question. If he hadn't, I would have been prepared to butt in and tell Whelan that Kang had only a few minutes left before he had to run off to a meeting. That would have been my signal to Kang that he had to wrap up the interview as soon as possible.

I breathed another sigh of relief when I read Whelan's story. It made no mention of that exchange.

We also got lucky with the *WSJ* story, co-written by Laura Meckler and Vanessa Fuhrmans, another influential reporter I had worked especially hard to cultivate a good relationship with.

The first paragraph of the story, which appeared on the front page on January 7, was close to perfect from our point of view: "John Edwards has been bashing big health insurers in recent days with the story of a girl who died waiting for a liver transplant. But the details of the case suggest the Democratic presidential candidate may be over-simplifying the tale."

The *Journal* reporters also reached out to AHIP's Ignagni, who told them that AHIP planned to work with medical societies on how to finance or cover experimental treatments. "We're not taking a PR approach to this but a policy approach," she said. "People want us to solve the problem, not just discuss it."

One of APCO's biggest successes came on January 11 when the *WSJ* ran an op-ed by Scott Gottlieb, a resident fellow at the American Enterprise Institute. Using John Edwards as his foil, Gottlieb opened with a glaring misrepresentation of Edwards's health care reform proposal and managed to work in a reference to Edwards's former career as a plaintiff's attorney, sure to raise the hackles of the *WSJ*'s conservative readers.

"Campaigning in the primaries," Gottlieb wrote, "former Sen. John Edwards is leveraging the tragic story of Nataline Sarkisyan—the 17-year-old California woman who recently died awaiting a liver transplant—to press his political attack on insurance companies and argue for European-style, single-payer health care. But the former trial lawyer, accustomed to using anecdotes of human suffering to frame his rhetoric, is twisting the facts."

Calling Edwards a single-payer supporter was such a stretch of the candidate's position that Gottlieb and the *Journal*'s op-ed page editors surely knew better. Edwards's platform—which was easy to find on his campaign Web site—actually called for *more* competition among private insurance companies, not their abolition under a government-run single-payer system.

The *WSJ* also gave Gottlieb ample space to include every key message CIGNA and AHIP could have wished for in the op-ed. It was a perfect example of how PR uses friendly pundits to shift the focus of news coverage away from a company under attack and toward a broader issue, and to create a new villain.

The real bad actor in this sad story, according to Gottlieb, was not CIGNA but someone of a type that a majority of the people who read the *WSJ*'s editorial pages loved to hate. In this case, it was—as characterized by Gottlieb—liberal, Europe-loving trial lawyer John Edwards.

THIS TIME, I SPIN MYSELF

Seeing the result of APCO's work was what finally got me to do what I knew I had to do but, until then, hadn't had the courage or will to do: quit my job.

It became clearer to me than ever that I was part of an industry that would do whatever it took to perpetuate its extraordinarily profitable existence.

I was dismayed with what I read and disgusted with myself. It finally dawned on me that, in my own quest for money and prestige, I had sold my soul. I had become the antithesis of what I had once tried to be as a journalist many years before. "Who are you?" I remember asking myself that day. "How did you get here? How did this happen to you?"

I had started hating my job before then, but never enough to walk away from it. I knew now I had had enough.

A few weeks earlier, I'd happened to be watching CBS's *Sunday Morning* when it aired a story about people who had left corporate jobs late in their careers to do something that paid less but gave them a greater sense that they were engaging in "right livelihood," as the Buddha would say. One of the people interviewed was Margie Maxwell, a CIGNA colleague who, I learned to my surprise, had left her high-paying job as vice president of sales in the Carolinas to become the director of development at a clinic that provided free health care to the poor.

Maxwell flashed back to mind after I read Gottlieb's op-ed, so I tracked her down to find out how things were working out for her. She told me she was making a fraction of what she had made at CIGNA, but she had never been happier. I confided to her that I wanted to leave CIGNA, too, but I didn't have the guts to do it—and I didn't have any idea how I would earn a living if I did.

"Well, Wendell," she said. "You're just going to have to leap and trust that the net will appear—because it will."

Hokey as it sounds, I decided the universe was telling me what I needed to hear through Maxwell, so I made up my mind that day. I was going to go into a new line of work. I just didn't know what it would be.

There's a reason I couldn't get Maxwell's advice out of my head: I was stone sober. In previous years, I would have been consuming enough alcohol to stay sufficiently anesthetized. But I had quit drinking—on October 17, 2006, to be exact—after coming to the conclusion that I was slowly committing suicide by drinking at least a six-pack of beer almost every single night to keep from thinking and feeling. Even when I was buzzed, though, I couldn't get out of my head the nagging belief that I was put on this earth to do something much more important than what I had been doing for the last twenty years. I didn't have a clue what it might be, but I decided that I would never find out if I kept destroying my own liver.

I'm confident that if I had not quit drinking, I would not have been affected by *Sicko* the way I had been, and I probably would not even have thought about going to the RAM expedition in the first place. I also doubt that I would have allowed myself to get so emotionally involved in the life and death of Nataline Sarkisyan.

A few days after talking to Maxwell and after many conversations with my family—and with their support—I asked my department's HR director if she could come to my office to discuss a personnel matter. I was going to take the leap.

My boss was not shocked when the HR director told her that I wanted to leave. A few weeks earlier, during one of our one-on-one meetings, Petren had seemed exasperated that I was not contributing as much as she thought I should.

"Wendell, you don't seem to be engaged," she said to me.

I made an effort to assure her that I was, indeed, engaged—but she and I both knew the truth.

Not only was I no longer "engaged" in my responsibilities as chief flack for the company, but I also didn't see eye to eye with her or Hanway on health care reform, and I had simply had it with trying to "protect, defend and enhance" the company's reputation. I didn't have it in me to handle any more horror stories. Nataline Sarkisyan's life and death had affected me profoundly.

Petren accepted my decision to leave but asked me to stay on for several more weeks. She needed time to determine who would assume my responsibilities, and she wanted me to stay long enough to help with the company's annual meeting of shareholders, which would be held in April, and the first-quarter earnings report, which would be released on May 1.

I agreed.

My last day as a CIGNA employee was May 2, 2008, the day after we announced that we had earned $265 million, or ninety-four cents a share, on revenues of $4.6 billion during the first three months of the year. The stock price closed that afternoon on the New York Stock Exchange at $42.26, up 3.5 percent from the day before.

CIGNA had had a very good day on Wall Street. Investors were happy because CIGNA had exceeded their expectations. CIGNA executives on the lead team, all of whom had stock options—me included—were richer financially.

But I was richer in every way thinkable.

CHAPTER IX

ERISA Stymies the Sarkisyans, and Us

WHILE CIGNA rightfully worried about the public relations black eye it might get as a result of the Sarkisyan case, the company's lawyers had no such concern that the Sarkisyan family's lawyer, Mark Geragos, could bring successful criminal or civil charges against the company.

Brian Benjet (who headed litigation for CIGNA) hired attorney Debra Yang out of an abundance of caution. He wanted to have a well-known L.A. attorney with a high-powered law firm ready to rumble in the unlikely event that her successor in the U.S. Attorney's Office charged CIGNA with murder. He knew, though, that she would probably never be needed, at least not in a courtroom. There was no reason to spend much time worrying that Ed Hanway would go to jail—or that the company would ever have to pay the Sarkisyans a dime.

The reason was that CIGNA had federal law on its side—as the unintended consequence of something that most attorneys and patients know little about. And the reason that so few people know about it is because, as important as it is, most reporters haven't figured out how to write about it in ways that their readers—or even their editors—can understand. I know because whenever I tried to explain the law to reporters—or anyone else, for that matter—I couldn't do it well enough to keep eyes from glazing over. It defies being reduced to a sound bite. Trust me, though: It's something that very likely pertains to you—and could be a factor in whether you have success in the courts if you ever think you have good reason to sue your employer or insurer over a coverage decision. So please stay with me.

In the early 1970s, an alarming number of retiring workers were getting the often-devastating news that they would not be receiving the retirement benefits promised by their employers. To protect employees' pensions, Congress passed the Employee Retirement Income Security Act of 1974, better known by its acronym, ERISA. Under ERISA, employers must fund pension plans sufficiently so they will be able to pay out promised benefits when their employees retire, and they must keep the pension money separate from other company funds and held in a trust. By doing this, the funds will be protected even if a company declares bankruptcy.

As North Carolina attorney and ERISA expert Brent Adams wrote in a blog post soon after Nataline died, members of Congress had good intentions when they passed the law, believing that beneficiaries of the law would be workers, not employers. "The legislation . . . [was] a well-intentioned law that Congress passed in large part to address the theft of employee retirement benefits by corporations in the Rust Belt which were going broke," Adams wrote. "Executives of these corporations were stealing money from employee pension plans, and longtime dedicated employees reached their retirement age only to find that their hard-earned pension benefits had been stolen by the corporate bosses."

While the motivation of Congress was to protect employer-sponsored pension plans, federal courts over the years have interpreted the law to apply to *all* employee benefits, including health plans. That wouldn't be so bad if the law just pertained to the solvency of the health plans. The problem for many people is that it goes much further. Because it is a federal law, ERISA preempts state laws—meaning that employer-sponsored plans are largely exempt from state benefit mandates and consumer protections. As a consequence, state insurance commissioners have almost no regulatory authority over ERISA-protected plans. Additionally, the 130 million Americans enrolled in ERISA-protected plans cannot sue their insurance company or employer in state court if they have been denied coverage for a treatment or procedure—as Nataline was. They can attempt to sue in federal court, but the potential remedies are so limited by the law that plaintiffs often have trouble even getting a lawyer to take their cases. There are relatively few lawyers who specialize in ERISA cases or are even knowledgeable of how the law affects health benefits.

The Sarkisyans had never heard of ERISA before Nataline died. In fact, it was not until the day after she died that the Sarkisyans and their attorney learned that the family's insurance plan was protected by ERISA.

"When we first started working on the Sarkisyan case, our objective was to get her that liver transplant," said Tamar Arminak, the lawyer at Geragos & Geragos who did most of the legal work for the family. "ERISA was not yet on our minds. Nataline died on a Thursday night, and Friday morning we realized Mr. Sarkisyan's plan was covered under ERISA. We were familiar with ERISA but thought obviously that a situation like this would be exempt from ERISA protections. I discovered quickly that it wasn't."

Hilda Sarkisyan's main mission in life today is to make people aware of the law and how it can affect them, and to get Congress to change it. In her view, it allows insurance companies to literally get away with murder. Sarkisyan has many members of Congress and most state insurance commissioners on her side. But she also has a familiar and very powerful opponent: CIGNA and its fellow insurance companies.

Insurers and their big-business allies are adamantly opposed to any changes in the law. So important is ERISA's protection that CIGNA and other big for-profit insurers joined several of the country's largest employers—coincidentally, less than a month before Nataline died—to bankroll a front group called the National Coalition on Benefits. The sole purpose of the coalition is to fight any attempt to tinker with ERISA. They like ERISA for the very same reasons that state insurance regulators, consumer advocates, and many jurists don't: It allows insurers to thumb their noses at state laws designed to protect consumers against insurance company abuses.

As the National Association of Insurance Commissioners noted in a comprehensive report on the often harmful consequence to consumers of ERISA's preemption of state laws, "ERISA provides few rights to consumers and, more significantly, it is used as a weapon to block the states' implementation of health care consumer rights."[1]

One of the reasons big employers are so fiercely protective of ERISA is that it allows companies with facilities in more than one state to offer uniform benefit packages to their employees whether they work in Portland, Oregon, or Portland, Maine. Companies can administer their employee benefit plans more easily and less expensively because—thanks to ERISA—they do not have to comply with varying state insurance regulations and consumer protections. However, as important as that is to both employers and their insurance companies—such as Grigor Sarkisyan's employer, Mercedes-Benz, and CIGNA—even more important is the near-total shield that ERISA provides them, preventing them from being sued.

Because of ERISA, Geragos could not sue CIGNA in any California state court for refusing to pay for Nataline's transplant. But he could not bring suit against CIGNA in federal court, either, because—believe it or not—Nataline died. Few lawyers sue insurers in federal court because, under ERISA, the only remedy their clients are entitled to receive—even if a judge and jury agree they've been wronged—are the costs the insurer refused to cover. The law does not allow federal judges or juries to award punitive damages, so they cannot order an insurer to provide any compensation for pain, suffering, or lost wages. Further, if the patient who was denied coverage dies, the insurer cannot be ordered to pay anything to the patient's survivors.

Because of this shield of protection, insurers have no financial
incentive to provide timely treatment, wrote Jamie Court, president of
Consumer Watchdog, in his 1999 book, *Making a Killing* (co-written
with Francis Smith):

> And that is the good news. The bad news is that companies are
> obligated to provide the cost of the benefit only when the patient
> survives long enough to receive it. If the patient dies before receiv-
> ing the treatment, the insurer or HMO pays nothing. Because there
> is no meaningful penalty for denying medically necessary treat-
> ment, there is no incentive to approve costly care.
>
> Imagine that the penalty for bank robbery was limited to
> giving back the stolen money. No jail time, no fines, just pay the
> money back—and only if you are caught. To top it off, the repaid
> money would be interest free. Would bank robbery increase under
> such circumstances? That's the situation HMOs and insurers enjoy
> under ERISA.[2]

In his blog post headlined "Mark Geragos Is Wasting His Time,"
ERISA expert Adams wrote:

> The general public does not understand that if they are in a
> dispute with a health insurance company that is governed by
> ERISA, as most [employer-based] plans are, the insurance com-
> pany itself gets to decide whether it should have to pay for health
> insurance benefits. The federal court will not intervene to help
> these unfortunate employees and their families who desperately
> need health insurance benefits. The federal courts will only reverse
> the insurance companies if the courts find that the insurance
> companies have "abused their discretion" in denying benefits. In
> layman's terms, what this means is if there is any evidence whatso-
> ever to support an insurance company's denial of benefits, the
> federal judges will turn their head and ignore this injustice . . .

Never mind that the denial of claims goes straight to the bottom line of insurance companies' profits.

ANOTHER REASON FOR THE MANAGED CARE BACKLASH

ERISA's harmful consequences to consumers were not nearly as much of a concern back in the day when most Americans were enrolled in indemnity plans. All that changed when employers—at the urging of insurance companies—began herding their employees into HMOs and other managed care plans in the 1990s.

As Karl Polzer, senior researcher at the George Washington University's National Health Policy Forum, and Pat Butler, a lawyer and policy analyst, wrote in *Health Affairs*, "ERISA's limited remedies for injuries can be more damaging to consumers when a managed care plan refuses coverage than when an indemnity plan refuses payment because managed care plan denials occur *before* treatment, whereas indemnity plan disputes typically occur *after* care has been rendered."[3] (Emphasis added.)

The only way to correct what Adams called a "ridiculous perversion of the law" is for Congress to change ERISA. Supreme Court justice Ruth Bader Ginsburg is among many in the legal world who agree that ERISA should be reexamined. In a 2004 opinion, she concurred that ERISA "completely preempted" a Texas law that sought to allow participants in group plans to sue their HMOs for refusing to pay for a doctor-recommended treatment. But Ginsburg added that she was joining "the rising judicial chorus urging that Congress and this Court revisit what is an unjust and increasingly tangled ERISA regime."

Another judge who expressed concern about ERISA was Judge Gary Feess of the District Court for the Central District of California, who because of the law had no alternative but to dismiss a breach-of-contract suit brought by the Sarkisyans against CIGNA. In ruling on April 16, 2009, Feess wrote that "in reaching this conclusion, the Court is mindful of the possibility that a finding of ERISA preemption may ultimately deprive Plaintiffs of a meaningful remedy for CIGNA's denial of coverage, even if wrongful, because the benefits are no longer necessary in view of Nataline's death, and because extra-contractual, compensatory, and punitive damages are not available under ERISA. This is an unfortunate consequence of the compromise Congress made in enacting ERISA, but it cannot preclude a finding of preemption."

One of the plaintiffs in the Supreme Court case that challenged the scope of the Texas law was CIGNA, which was so confident that the justices would agree with it that it was willing to risk taking the case to the high court for a definitive ruling. A win would mean a great deal to the industry because it would discourage future lawsuits against insurers and employers.

The case reached the Supreme Court when CIGNA appealed a lower-court ruling that sided with a CIGNA health-plan member, Ruby Calad, who'd sued CIGNA in state court in Texas after being sent home from the hospital—against her doctor's orders—the day after a complicated hysterectomy. A CIGNA nurse told Calad that the company would not pay for an additional day in the hospital because she didn't meet CIGNA's criteria for a longer stay. She went home but had to return to the hospital soon for further treatment.

In its unanimous decision in the case (*CIGNA HealthCare of Texas, Inc. v. Calad et al.*), the Supreme Court ruled that CIGNA's refusal to pay for a longer stay in the hospital was a "benefit eligibility decision" rather than a medical-treatment decision. The consequence of the ruling was that Calad could not pursue her case against CIGNA in state court, where she could have been awarded punitive damages. Her lawsuit would have to be transferred to federal court and be subject to the restricted remedies provided under ERISA.

Corporate America and the insurance industry breathed a collective sigh of relief when the ruling was announced. Industry executives had known that whatever the final ruling turned out to be, it would have long-term ramifications for employer-sponsored plans—and insurance company profits.

The ruling in CIGNA's favor was a big setback for consumer advocates, but my job was to spin the decision as a major win for consumers. I decided that the way to do that was to argue that ERISA helped employers and health plans keep coverage affordable.

So I wrote in a June 21, 2004, statement that ERISA "has for many years helped ensure that participants in health benefit plans have numerous protections, including access to quick resolution of any coverage disputes through internal and external appeals processes. By providing consistent standards for the administration of health plans, ERISA also has helped employers provide health care benefits for their employees at a reasonable cost."

I went on to suggest that there was no need for health-plan enrollees to be able to sue CIGNA in state court because it had a "fair, efficient and equitable" appeals process in place to address any concerns that anyone might have regarding coverage interpretations. "Today's decision," I concluded, "supports this approach."

The Sarkisyans viewed the CIGNA process quite differently. They certainly did not agree that it was fair, efficient, or equitable.

DON'T HOLD YOUR BREATH FOR CONGRESS TO CHANGE ERISA

Passing a 2,407-page health care reform bill has proved easier for Congress than amending ERISA, so far. The problem, of course, is that every time a member of Congress tries to change the law, big insurance and big business swing into action, pouring millions of dollars into public relations and advertising campaigns.

In 1998, when Senator Ted Kennedy (D-Mass.) and Representative John Dingell (D-Mich.) introduced a bill that would strip employers and insurers of their ERISA protections, the insurance industry launched another successful fearmongering campaign. The Health Insurance Association of America, one of AHIP's predecessors, quickly commissioned an actuarial analysis that predicted that 160,000 people would lose their coverage because businesses, fearing costly legal settlements, would stop offering health care benefits. The fearmongering worked—and has worked every time ERISA has been under attack.

The National Coalition on Benefits (NCB), formed in 2007, was not the first group of its kind that the insurance industry had funded, at least in part, to defeat attempts to weaken ERISA. As noted earlier, they pooled resources in the late 1990s to pay the big PR firm Porter Novelli to create and run the Health Benefits Coalition, which had the same goal: protecting ERISA. The HBC helped scare members of Congress and their constituents away from the Patient's Bill of Rights that Dingell had cosponsored with Representative Charles Norwood Jr. (D-Ga.). Like the Kennedy-Dingell bill, the Patient's Bill of Rights would have allowed people enrolled in employer-sponsored plans to sue their insurers in state courts.

The HBC allied with the conservative group FreedomWorks to demonize the bill. FreedomWorks warned in a 1999 press release that the bill would "only take money out of consumers' checkbooks and put it into the pockets of trial lawyers, making health insurance less affordable for all Americans." Congress never passed a Patient's Bill of Rights because the House and the Senate, which had passed different versions of the legislation, could never resolve their differences.

As Congress geared up for the health care reform debate in 2007, insurers and their big-employer customers launched the HBC's successor, the NCB, to once again scare lawmakers away from changing ERISA in any meaningful way. The coalition's key message: "Don't erode what works to fix what's broken."

Representative Dennis Kucinich (D-Ohio) tried to amend the 2010 reform bill to change ERISA, but his amendment died after the U.S. Chamber of Commerce warned House leaders that it would oppose the entire bill if it included the ERISA amendment. While many provisions of the 2010 reform bill will apply to all insurance plans, including employer-sponsored plans, it keeps the ERISA protections for insurers and employers intact.

Still, Hilda Sarkisyan has no intention of backing down.

In 2008, with help from family and friends, she organized Nataline's Legacy Fashion Show to raise money "to stop for-profit insurance companies from being allowed to decide who gets to live and who gets to die."

They decided to do a fashion show—and to hold it every year on or near Nataline's July 10 birthday—because of her dream of being a fashion designer.[4]

"We found drawings of twenty-two gowns in Nataline's room," said Sarkisyan. "My daughter wanted to go to the Fashion Institute of Design after she graduated from high school." At the second annual show, in 2009 (which attracted nearly five hundred people to the showroom of the Mercedes-Benz dealership in Calabasas, where Nataline's father still worked), Beverly Hills haute couture designer Pol' Atteu, himself an Armenian American, brought one of Nataline's designs to life.

A story in the *Armenian Reporter* newspaper—covering the 2009 fashion show and the Sarkisyans' battle with CIGNA—quoted Hilda Sarkisyan as saying, "CIGNA insurance denied my daughter the liver transplant she needed and I lost her. But I'm not going to let this go. I'm not going to let insurance companies get away with murder again. I don't want Nataline's death to be in vain."

I was mentioned in that same newspaper story: "CIGNA's disastrous decision even prompted a high-ranking company executive to resign. The CIGNA official who quit told CNN that CIGNA's decision about Nataline prompted him to walk away with disgust and pursue health care reform on Capitol Hill."

I finally met the Sarkisyan family in their home in January 2009, six months after the second fashion show. An NBC *Dateline* crew was there to film what turned out to be a tense and emotional but ultimately cordial meeting. Before I left, I promised the Sarkisyans that I would help them in their campaign to change ERISA.

This book is a start.

CHAPTER X

A Victory, of Sorts

AFTER nearly a century of failed attempts to enact universal health care, everyone knew that the fight that began when Barack Obama took office would be arduous. I knew better than most, but even I didn't foresee the ferocious warfare we would endure for more than a year.

The struggle eventually did put our country on a new path toward remedying injustice in health care. But thanks to the shrewd and well-funded operatives of the health insurance industry and its allies, not one inch of this ground was gained without political turmoil.

Obama's election in 2008 electrified the nation and much of the world. It left him well positioned to take on the big challenges if he acted quickly, and he wasted no time. Even as he moved into the White House pushing a stimulus bill to counter the economic disaster created by the collapse of investment banks and other financial institutions, his staff geared up for a quick start on health care reform.

His opponents portray him as a "socialist" and a "radical," but in truth Obama is not even a hard-core liberal. He is a moderate centrist who often leans to the left. He may be socially liberal when it comes to reform—he once said that if we could start from scratch, he would

support a publicly financed single-payer system—but he is also a prag-
matist who understands the political realities of Washington.

Obama rose to power partly on the strength of his ability to adapt
to different audiences. "My experience being able to walk into a public-
housing development and turn around and walk into a corporate boardroom and communicate effectively in either venue means that I'm
more likely to be able to build the kinds of coalitions and craft the sort
of message that appeals to a broad range of people," he said in a 2000
interview.[1]

Obama's fervent supporters often thought they heard more than
they really did. Still, his 2008 campaign promises about health care
were fairly clear. Crafted with the help of Harvard economist David
Cutler, Obama's original plan called for employer mandates, federal
coverage of catastrophic-care costs, and tax credits to help low- and
middle-income families afford private health insurance. As I noted
previously, he opposed any requirement that everyone buy insurance,
one of the few points on which he disagreed with rival Hillary Clinton. His platform also called for the creation of a public health plan to
compete with private insurers—as did Clinton's and that of his other
early opponent, John Edwards—but Obama never promised to fall
on his sword for a government-run plan.[2]

In the end, Obama produced a legislative victory that will accomplish much of what the Clintons had hoped for in their earlier effort:
expanded coverage and controlled costs. It will add sixteen million
people to state Medicaid programs through expanded eligibility rules.
It will offer tax credits to about sixteen million more people in families
earning up to 400 percent of the federal poverty level (about $88,000
for a family of four). And, according to the Congressional Budget
Office (CBO), it will reduce the federal deficit by $143 billion over
ten years.

The legislation falls short in other respects—most disappoint-
ingly in that it does not include a government-run public option to
compete with private insurers. But politics is the art of the possible, as

Otto von Bismarck said, and in the end, President Obama and his chief of staff, Rahm Emanuel, calculated that sacrificing the public option was a price worth paying to nail down other significant gains in the bill.

Obama's victory is really just a pit stop in an ongoing, contentious battle that split the country wide open while showcasing the skill of corporate America at getting what it wants in a white-hot, polarized media and political environment. The stakes were high, and clashes over health care reform erupted in every corner of the nation, opening wounds and reviving tribal grudges from generations ago, like a dormant volcano brought back to life.

Health insurers and other special interests opened their pocketbooks to frustrate reform and protect huge profit streams. Political front groups flourished, nurtured with millions of dollars from shadowy corporate sponsors, including insurers. Powerful images and words were unleashed. Antireform operatives concocted myths, libeled Democratic leaders, used racist slogans and pictures, and questioned the patriotism of people supporting a just health care system. Fox News eagerly broadcast these antics and messages—morning, noon, and night. And, perhaps most important, the health insurance industry showered members of Congress with political contributions—and overwhelmed them with thousands of lobbyists to push its propaganda.

Guided by professional political organizers with deep roots in the Republican Party and the lobbying world, notably former House majority leader Dick Armey of Texas, opponents of health care reform mounted shrill protests that led to the formation of the Tea Party. The GOP made the political calculation that killing health care reform—at least as envisioned by the Democrats—was its leading hope of regaining power. This belief was crystallized in a quote from Senator Jim DeMint (R-S.C.), who said that the defeat of the initiative would be Obama's "Waterloo."

Opponents were handed the first round when Obama tapped

former Senate majority leader Tom Daschle of South Dakota to be his
secretary of health and human services. He intended to put Daschle
in charge of health care reform, but this plan fell apart when Daschle
ran into difficulty in the Senate Finance Committee after the members learned he'd failed to report free use of limousine services offered by a corporate donor. Jokes flew about "limousine liberals," and
only weeks into the new administration Daschle withdrew from con-
sideration. It was merely the first speed bump Obama would hit on his
tortuous path to health care reform.

Obama recovered quickly, submitting his initial budget and saying
in a speech to Congress that health care reform was his number-one
legislative goal. He proposed the creation of a $634 billion health care
"reserve fund"—a down payment based on new taxes and savings, including cuts of Medicare subsidies to private insurers for optional managed care plans. Obama's initial plan outlined insurance coverage for
tens of millions of Americans while reining in fast-growing medical
costs that burdened middle- and lower-income families and strained
budgets at every level of government.[3]

His idea was to stimulate discussion among his Democratic allies
on Capitol Hill without being too detailed—a lesson from the Clinton
debacle sixteen years earlier. Unless he won congressional buy-in, he
thought, his plan would crash and burn, too. And sure enough, over the
next thirty days, Washington crackled with health care reform activity.

When Daschle asked that his nomination be withdrawn, Obama
replaced him with Kansas governor Kathleen Sebelius, who had had
that rare experience of successfully defying the health insurance industry.

When Obama officially kicked off the health care reform debate
with his March 5, 2009, summit—to which he invited more than
150 members of Congress, health-policy experts, and leaders of
groups representing doctors, hospitals, unions, big business, insurance
companies, and consumers—one of the people sitting in the East
Room was the health insurance industry's point person in Washington,

AHIP president Karen Ignagni. Ignagni's challenge was daunting, sort of like playing three-dimensional chess. She had to woo the media, deploy hundreds of lobbyists, enforce message discipline among the rich and powerful insurance CEOs on her board of directors, and generate impressive, "mediagenic" data—all while posing among gullible politicians as an honest broker. All these things she did, and in the process revised the public's archetype of a Washington insider—you don't have to be a round-faced, cigar-chomping, aging white man to be the capital's top lobbyist.

The soft-spoken Ignagni was the public face of an eight-hundred-billion-dollar-a-year industry, and her mission was to see health care reform passed that would benefit insurance company shareholders and executives and to help them avoid increased public accountability. For Ignagni, it was the biggest challenge in a career that had taken her on a remarkable path from protecting the health benefits of middle-class workers to protecting corporate titans who abused and overcharged their sick customers.

Ignagni grew up in Providence, Rhode Island, the child of a firefighter and a city hall worker. After graduating from Providence College in 1975 in the first class that included women, she was hired as a research analyst at the Social Security Administration. Two years later, she went to work for a group promoting national health insurance that was backed by Walter Reuther, the legendary president of the United Auto Workers. After two years, she joined the professional staff of Senator Claiborne Pell (D-R.I.) and worked on a panel that later became the Health, Education, Labor, and Pension (HELP) Committee. During her three years on Capitol Hill, Ignagni often worked with the staff of Senator Ted Kennedy, the nation's leading advocate of universal coverage.

While working for Pell, a social liberal and a labor favorite, Ignagni came to the attention of the AFL-CIO, and the huge labor federation hired her in 1982. For eleven years, she worked on pensions and health care, rising to director of the health benefits department, which served more than eleven million members. She reportedly spent much of her time helping negotiate new managed care plans.[4] During this period, she also completed an executive MBA program at Loyola University, in Baltimore.

In 1993, a headhunting firm recruited Ignagni to be the president of the Group Health Association of America (later renamed the American Association of Health Plans, or AAHP). Suddenly, she turned her back on years of progressive politics and became the leader of one of two rival trade groups that would eventually merge to make AHIP. Her first job was successfully fending off President Clinton's Health Security initiative.

As you may recall, a headhunter also recruited me to my new job at CIGNA in 1993, and I would work with Ignagni on the same side of many battles for the next fifteen years. Not only were we allies in the fight against the Clinton plan, but we were also allies in subsequent fights with lawmakers (who tried for years to pass a Patient's Bill of Rights) and lawyers (who tried to force managed care companies to deal more fairly with both patients and their doctors). I also worked closely with her communications team in developing PR plans and talking points and coordinating countless media interviews.

Ignagni quickly made a name for herself. She was frequently listed among the "top guns" and most influential lobbyists in Washington. In 2003, when AAHP merged with the Health Insurance Association of America to form AHIP, Ignagni prevailed over HIAA's Chip Kahn to become CEO of the new group. Her compensation soared to $1.94 million in 2008,[5] up from $400,000 in 1998.[6]

Within months after Obama's White House summit, AHIP, despite Ignagni's promise to help the president pass health care reform, unleashed its sophisticated, multipronged attack to undermine it. The relationship between the White House and the industry changed from cordial and collaborative to hostile when it became clear to Obama and his reform team that AHIP was conducting a duplicitous campaign— saying one thing and doing another. Instead of further pledges of

cooperation from the industry, the American people got fearmongering, misleading ads, coordinated attacks by conservative opinion col-
umnists and health-policy experts for hire, deceptive studies and
reports, and front groups that ran antireform ads or orchestrated Tea
Party events, funded at least in part by insurers.

From 2007 to mid-2009, insurance and HMO political contributions and lobbying expenses totaled a jaw-dropping $586 million,
according to Public Campaign. At the height of the battle, the industries were spending nearly $700,000 a day to influence the political
process.[7]

The key goals of health care reform—and the battle lines—had
been delineated by the end of March 2009. Top House Democrats
pledged to pass a health care bill before the August recess. Democrats
also favored reserving the right to use a common parliamentary budget maneuver called "reconciliation" to pass the bill in the Senate by
majority vote rather than the sixty votes needed to block a filibuster.
But Senator Max Baucus (D-Mont.), chairman of the Finance Committee, and Senator Kent Conrad (D-N.Dak.), chairman of the Budget Committee, said they opposed reconciliation, preferring to find
the necessary votes from the GOP side to get the sixty supporters
needed.

House leaders reached consensus on the creation of a public
option—vehemently opposed by insurers and Republicans—to function as an instant, formidable competitor in the reformed health insurance marketplace. The public option was the brainchild of Yale political
science professor Jacob Hacker, whose arguments were detailed and
compelling.[8] Progressive activists, labor unions, and their umbrella
group, Health Care for America Now (HCAN), embraced the public
option as the only way to force millions of new customers to buy health
insurance without creating a public backlash. Only if Americans were
allowed to choose such a plan would there be broad public acceptance
of the compulsory purchase of health insurance, they argued, and polls
consistently backed them up.[9]

It was an article of faith among liberals that a national public option would be the best way to curb soaring health care costs. The most prominent public plan, Medicare, had recorded annual spending growth significantly lower than private insurers' over the previous decade, with per capita costs growing by 4.4 percent a year under Medicare versus 7.4 percent under private health insurance.[10] But this superior cost-control performance was exactly why so many health care providers, from drugmakers to doctors and hospitals, were leery of health care reform. They all worried that a public option would underpay them and take away their power to charge what the traffic would bear—as they had long complained that Medicare did. The drug and hospital industries eventually cut deals with Obama that locked in limits on their own health care reform concessions (in return for their not attacking reform).

Meanwhile, insurers worried—and rightfully so—that they would fail to compete against the superior provider networks, lower overhead, and lower premiums of a public option. And, a government-operated plan wouldn't concern itself with surging insurance company profits and obscene executive pay, focusing instead on processing claims efficiently and setting reasonable rules on what services were covered.

In the ensuing war, one of the most impressive and well-planned early maneuvers of Ignagni and her industry was performed by United-Health Group, which in 2007—just as the political stars were aligning for health care reform—had bought its own think tank. The Lewin Group, a respected health-policy consulting firm in northern Virginia that had been working with governments and industry for forty years, became a wholly owned unit of a UnitedHealth subsidiary, Ingenix. A credible source of economic data and analysis in the health care arena, Lewin was now tarred with a perceived conflict of interest. John Sheils, a vice president, tried to limit damage by proclaiming Lewin's editorial independence from UnitedHealth, but that didn't square with its later conduct.

In April 2009, just as it became apparent that the public option

was being seriously considered by Democratic leadership, Lewin released a report claiming that a public option would force 119 million
Americans out of their employer-sponsored health plans and into the
government insurance plan. Republicans eagerly embraced the claim,
which, as it turned out, wasn't based on any specific legislation. Nevertheless, House minority whip Eric Cantor of Virginia used the data to
bolster Republicans' claims that the public option would doom the
country's employer-based health care system.

A July 23, 2009, story in the *Washington Post* pointed out how
ridiculous that framing was.[11] The story even quoted a Lewin vice
president acknowledging that Americans would not be forced into a
government-run plan if a public option were created and that many
people "might very well be better off" if they could choose between a
government-run plan and private options. After its analysis had been
widely questioned, Lewin reduced its estimate of the impact of the
public option, saying that "only" 88.1 million people would shift from
employer-based coverage to the public option under the Democrats'
plan—whereas in late July the nonpartisan CBO found that the public
option would draw only 11 million people from the 170 million covered by private health plans. That didn't keep opponents from continuing to use Lewin's disputed public option projections as supporting
evidence that Obama and congressional leaders were bent on "a government takeover" of the health care system that would lead to long
waits to see a doctor, care denied by government bureaucrats, and
huge tax increases.

The industry also used its vast information technology resources
to provide "helpful" actuarial data to its friends. Virtually no one on
Capitol Hill had the background or skills to question this evidence.
Congressional staffers at the highest levels of the discussions confessed that they had to ask insurance companies themselves for
comparative actuarial analyses of various scenarios to help formulate
proposals for members of Congress. What else could they do? Not
having access to the actual data, congressional offices couldn't run

such research independently. *BusinessWeek* captured the effectiveness of that approach in a cover story on August 6, 2009, which noted,

> The carriers have succeeded in redefining the terms of the reform debate to such a degree that no matter what specifics emerge in the voluminous bill Congress may send to President Obama this fall, the insurance industry will emerge more profitable. Health reform could come with a $1 trillion price tag over the next decade, and it may complicate matters for some large employers. But insurance CEOs ought to be smiling . . .
>
> The industry has already accomplished its main goal of at least curbing, and maybe blocking altogether, any new publicly administered insurance program that could grab market share from the corporations that dominate the business. UnitedHealth has distinguished itself by more deftly and aggressively feeding sophisticated pricing and actuarial data to information-starved congressional staff members. With its rivals, the carrier has also achieved a secondary aim of constraining the new benefits that will become available to tens of millions of people who are currently uninsured. That will make the new customers more lucrative to the industry.[12]

Leading the fight against such overwhelming industry resources was HCAN, which had been launched in the summer of 2008 for the purpose of winning meaningful health care reform. HCAN ultimately comprised more than one thousand member organizations, including the nation's biggest unions, civil rights groups, and progressive political organizations. HCAN would spend forty-seven million dollars in the battle, with its money coming from its members and grants from foundations. Atlantic Philanthropies was its biggest funder. Although they couldn't compete with the money available to insurers and their allies, progressives were determined not to get steamrolled the way they had in 1993.

Led by Richard Kirsch, a veteran organizer and political activist from New York, HCAN emerged as a focal point with local activist organizations under contract in forty-four states. "We represent the deepest single-issue coalition in modern American history," said Jeff Blum, HCAN co-chairman and director of USAction, a leading progressive grassroots organization. Blum and Kirsch conceived of HCAN as a way to win universal coverage by enlisting local activists, providing them with solid funding and research, giving them continuous advice on how to exert influence, and running targeted television ad campaigns in their states.

Blum and Kirsch started by recruiting the Service Employees International Union (SEIU) and the American Federation of State, County and Municipal Employees (AFSCME), each representing large numbers of health care workers. When HCAN debuted, the steering committee included unions, community groups, physician groups, and the influential Center for American Progress, seen by many as a Democratic shadow government before Obama's inauguration. CAP president John Podesta led Obama's transition team.

When AHIP staked out its "pro-reform" position in December 2008, it proposed the acceptance by insurers of all customers regardless of medical history and the cessation of canceling customers' coverage when they got sick—but only if all Americans were required to buy coverage from private companies. The group did not suggest charging everyone in a given community the same prices, and thus its proposal would have left millions of sick or high-risk residents in constant danger of being charged whatever insurers wanted. Kirsch aimed to kill this proposal as quickly as possible.

All along, Kirsch knew that HCAN needed to embolden centrist Blue Dog Democrats, especially freshmen and conservative incumbents from districts where Obama had fared poorly in the election. In addition to buying millions of dollars of TV advertisements, HCAN planned to make use of an unprecedented progressive activist base with the help of coalition members such as the AFL-CIO, MoveOn.org,

SEIU, AFSCME, Americans United for Change, the Center for Community Change, the American Federation of Teachers, Campaign for America's Future, ACORN, True Majority, the United Food and Commercial Workers, USPIRG, and the Communications Workers of America.

"The vision from the beginning was to bring together the largest membership groups in the country to form a coalition that combines impact in Washington with a massive field presence across the country," said Kirsch. "We're part of a lot of coalitions, but HCAN is edgy in a unique way," said Lynda Tran of SEIU. "It has a 'street heat' that we're known for as well. The combination of grassroots and new media and online organizing gives it a special force and energy."[13]

The tactics were tried-and-true, including bringing delegations of HCAN field partners to district offices of members of Congress, flooding their offices with handwritten letters, arranging for leaders of local grassroots groups to visit members' offices in Washington, generating media coverage of protests and rallies, visiting newspaper editorial boards, releasing research reports, and organizing large-scale rallies in Washington. HCAN became a success because it adopted a coordination role that had never been used on the left as it had on the right.

One of the biggest conflicts among progressives was between advocates of a single-payer system, like those in Canada and Europe, and those who believed that the public option would have a more viable chance of getting through Congress. Single-payer supporters thought that HCAN had joined the corrupt Washington establishment when it accepted the public option as an alternative to a completely government-financed system after it became clear that Obama and congressional leaders were not interested in pursuing what they believed would be too radical a proposal for even many Democrats.

It was soon after Obama's March 5 summit—when the president and members of Congress seemed to be falling for Ignagni's pledge of cooperation—that I began, nervously, making calls to the few reform advocates I knew of to offer my help. I was paranoid at first, constantly worried that I would talk to someone who would mention what I was doing to someone who might have close ties to AHIP or CIGNA. Even though at the time no one outside of my family knew anything about what I was contemplating, I imagined that my phones were tapped and that my house was under surveillance. If the industry knew I was thinking about giving aid and comfort to the enemy, it would undoubtedly try to shut me up, I feared. I envisioned all kinds of ways they would try to do that. When the first calls didn't seem to get me anywhere, I almost gave up. But the more evidence I saw that the industry was behind the efforts to kill or eviscerate reform, the more determined I became to do something. I just didn't know what it would be—although I hoped I could do it anonymously.

Among the people I contacted were the PR staffers at the California Nurses Association. They were cordial when we met, but I never heard back from them. They clearly didn't see how I could help them. I searched the Internet for names of local health care reform advocates in Philadelphia. I met with one for lunch. We had a great conversation, and he offered to put me in touch with the leadership of Physicians for a National Health Program, one of the most prominent single-payer organizations in the country. They, too, were cordial but offered little help beyond their best wishes.

One of the first people to see the potential of what I could bring to the reform effort was Michael Morrill, who several months earlier had launched a group in Pennsylvania called Keystone Progress. Morrill, I soon found out, was extraordinarily well connected. I mentioned to him that I was thinking of going to a meeting in Washington in early April that was being hosted by the Herndon Alliance, which billed itself as a coalition of minority, faith, labor, advocacy, business, and health care provider organizations that shared a common goal of "affordable health care for all." A friend of a friend of a friend had put me in touch with Bob Crittenden, Herndon's founder, and Crittenden had invited me to attend the group's next meeting as an observer.

It turned out that Morrill knew some of the people who would be at the meeting, and he arranged for me to talk afterward with three or four whom he described as heavy hitters. He even drove down to D.C. from his home in Reading, Pennsylvania, to introduce me to them in person. The one person who seemed more than marginally interested in me was Jacki Schechner, HCAN's communications director.

When Schechner returned to her office, she mentioned meeting me to some of her colleagues. As fate would have it, one of them was a former reporter I had worked with when I was at CIGNA, Avram Goldstein, who had covered for-profit health insurers for Bloomberg News. He'd been one of the best of a handful of reporters who covered the industry, and I had enjoyed working with him. I'd lost track of him after leaving CIGNA, and I'd had no idea he had left Bloomberg to join HCAN as its research director.

A few days later, Goldstein arranged for me to meet Kirsch at the 30th Street Station in Philadelphia. Kirsch was heading to a meeting in New York but got off the train in Philly long enough for us to have a conversation about exactly what I could bring to the table. It was at that meeting that the idea of me testifying before Congress was first mentioned.

At the same time that I was talking with HCAN, I also began to get to know John Stauber, who in 1993 had started the Center for Media and Democracy in Wisconsin "to investigate and counter spin corporations, industries and government agencies." I had secretly admired the center's work even when I was at CIGNA. Stauber had always hoped he would someday meet a PR guy who was willing to "spill his guts," as he put it. After a thorough vetting that included a formal background check, Stauber invited me to join CMD as senior fellow on health care. I jumped at the chance. My duties would involve doing research and contributing to CMD's Web site. I would also write a blog on health care reform. I told Stauber that I thought I should stay in touch with HCAN, and he agreed, although he was not a big fan of the organization. He was among those who thought that HCAN had caved too soon on single payer.

My continuing conversations with HCAN led to a two-hour meeting in the Dirksen Senate Office Building in early June with the staff of the Oversight and Investigations Subcommittee of the Senate Commerce, Science, and Transportation Committee, which was chaired by Senator Jay Rockefeller (D-W. Va.). After another background check, this one by the U.S. Senate, I got a call from committee staff asking me if I would be willing to testify at a June 24 public hearing.

I agreed, after talking it over with my family. I knew our lives would change forever as soon as I finished my testimony; I just didn't know how. Once again, I imagined the worst that could happen. But I knew that if I didn't do it, I would always regret it. This was my chance to possibly make a difference. The time had arrived for me to leap.

With the possible exception of my wedding day, June 24, 2009, was the scariest day of my life. The committee staff had alerted the Capitol Hill press corps that I would be testifying, so I knew there would be at least some news coverage of what I had to say. Fortunately, I would be testifying as part of a three-person panel on the need for reform and also for health insurers to be required to be more transparent in their dealings with consumers. The other panelists were people I had heard of and respected: Karen Pollitz of Georgetown University's Health Policy Institute and Nancy Metcalf of *Consumer Reports*.

When the hearing ended and I stood up, reporters swarmed around me. My new life as a very public reform advocate and critic of the industry had begun. Over the coming months, I would testify before two other congressional committees; appear at two press conferences with House leaders, including Speaker Nancy Pelosi of California and House Rules Committee chairwoman Louise Slaughter (D.-N.Y.); meet separately with dozens of members of both the House and the Senate and with scores of Hill staffers; and travel to more than half the states for speaking engagements and interviews. My fears about retaliation from the industry proved to be groundless. My former colleagues decided that the best way to deal with me was to pretend I didn't exist.

They knew that acknowledging me and what I was saying would only give me more exposure.

Within a month after my first appearance before Congress, House leaders pushed a bill through three committees that included the public option and a surtax on high-income earners. To win the support of the more conservative Blue Dog Democrats, the leadership agreed to include certain tax exemptions for businesses. No Republicans voted for it in any of the committees.

Getting the legislation through the Senate was going to be even more of a challenge. Two relevant committees were considering health care reform bills. The Senate HELP Committee, chaired by Chris Dodd (D-Conn.), sitting in for a gravely ill Ted Kennedy, passed a bill that included the public option on a party-line vote, 13–10. But Baucus was determined to keep the public option out of his Finance Committee bill. Regarded with suspicion by progressives, Baucus departed from Senate tradition by creating a working group of three Republican and three Democratic committee members to hold private meetings and forge a consensus on health care reform. The meetings dragged on for many weeks, raising suspicions that the Democrats were being duped by Republicans into believing that bipartisanship was achievable.

But progressives kept moving forward, and the American Medical Association, a crucial interest group, endorsed the public option—a far cry from its historic positions that had helped defeat reform for more than a century.

The month of August was a painful one for pro-reform forces. Ignagni bluntly warned members of Congress not to blast her industry during the August recess. She told the Associated Press that if lawmakers used the recess to vilify insurers, "members of Congress will come back to Washington without a strong sense that health care reform is doable. And that would be a lost opportunity. We think health care reform is going to be won or lost in August."

Obama had begun talking by then about insurance company

abuses and record profits, and Pelosi went so far as to call insurers "villains." Ignagni responded by saying that "when polls are slipping, people turn to tried-and-true tactics."[14]

Members of Congress scattered to their states and districts during the recess, and health insurance industry allies were waiting. Many legislators were confronted at town hall meetings by angry crowds—sometimes exhibiting mob behavior—who expressed an almost inchoate outrage over health care reform. Few seemed well informed about the policies they were protesting. At one event, several angry objectors carried signs demanding that the government keep its hands "off my Medicare," apparently not realizing that they were enrolled in the country's biggest government-run health care program.

I was a participant at one of these rowdy meetings and saw firsthand how angry and misinformed people were. Representative Bill Pascrell (D-N.J.) invited me to speak at a town hall he held at Montclair State University on September 3. More than a thousand people crammed into the auditorium, not so much to hear the speakers as to express their opinions. Reform opponents were on one side of the auditorium, and reform advocates were on the other side. I had to shout my remarks to be heard above the noise and chaos. Each side was determined to be louder than the other, so no one could hear anything being said.

Pascrell was able to calm the crowd long enough to conduct what he had hoped would be a Q&A session, but there were few questions. Most people just wanted to vent. One woman said she'd heard that some of the people working behind the scenes on the legislation had close ties to communists. Another woman said she'd heard that all the pizzeria owners in the area would be put out of business if health care reform legislation passed.

There was no doubt in my mind afterward that the insurance industry had played a role in what was clearly a well-orchestrated fear-mongering campaign—and a well-organized effort to get people out to disrupt the town halls.

Allies of the insurance industry had begun sending e-mails to millions of people with false claims about the contents of pending bills. One of the most insidious rumors was that the legislation would create government "death panels" to sort out which elderly people were too unhealthy or unworthy to get treatment through Medicare. Polls showed that millions of people, especially seniors, believed the rumors.

It was all part of a coordinated strategy. Journalists reported on memos from astroturf groups—like Dick Armey's FreedomWorks and Americans for Prosperity—that advised members on how to put congresspeople on the defensive by disrupting presentations and challenging everything they said in support of the Democrats' "socialist agenda." The objective was to make members of Congress believe that opposition to health care reform was widespread. Predictably, polls began to show that the public was buying into this manufactured imagery. HCAN responded by turning out thousands of people at hundreds of town hall meetings to physically position themselves to outmaneuver the Tea Party members and other reform opponents and blunt their media impact, but the damage had been done.

After the summer recess, Obama tried to restore support for reform by speaking to a rare joint session of Congress. In the September 9 speech, he criticized his opponents' "scare tactics" and made his strongest case yet for comprehensive reform. When Obama denied that illegal immigrants would be given health care coverage under any bill being considered by Congress, Representative Joe Wilson (R-S.C.) blurted out, "You lie!" Wilson was rebuked a week later by the House, and polls showed that Obama had stopped the slide in public opinion favoring reform.

Thanks to Pascrell, I was in the House gallery during the president's address—the first time I had been there since I'd left my job as a Washington correspondent thirty years earlier. Just being there was a moving experience, but to hear the president quote me (although not by name) was a spine-tingling moment. "As one former insurance executive testified before Congress," Obama said, "insurance companies are not only encouraged to find reasons to drop the seriously ill, they are rewarded for it. All of this is in service of meeting what this former executive called Wall Street's relentless profit expectations."

A week after the speech, Baucus finally gave up on his effort to win over any Republican members of his Finance Committee and introduced his long-awaited bill, which, to progressives' great disappointment, did not include a public option.

But shortly thereafter, in mid-October, the insurance industry made its first significant blunder. Insurers had insisted that Americans should face severe financial penalties if they did not buy health insurance. Unhappy that the penalties in the Baucus bill were not as significant as it had expected, AHIP hired PricewaterhouseCoopers (PWC) to produce a report showing that health care reform would hurt most Americans rather than help them. Touted by Ignagni in a conference call with reporters, the data showed that health care reform would drive premiums up for everyone—and that consumers would foot most of the bill for an excise tax on expensive health care plans. This was contrary to reports from the CBO and independent experts that concluded that insurance companies would respond to the tax by slowing the growth of health care costs.

White House staffers who had spent months trying to accommodate the industry's demands went ballistic, claiming that after months of respectful interaction, AHIP had blindsided them with a biased and purposely misleading report. "It comes on the eve of a vote that will reduce the industry's profits," White House spokeswoman Linda Douglass said. "It is hard to take it seriously. The analysis completely ignores critical policies that will lower costs for those who have insurance, expand coverage, and provide affordable health insurance options to millions of Americans who are priced out of today's health insurance market or are locked out by unfair insurance company practices."[15]

The firestorm became so intense that PWC backed away from its own findings, pointing out that it had focused only on the parts of health care reform that AHIP opposed, while ignoring everything else. "The disclaimer doesn't get PricewaterhouseCoopers entirely off the hook," wrote Ezra Klein in the *Washington Post*. "The methodological inadequacies of the report made the results nothing short of deceptive, and the final product still had PWC's name on it. But it makes it even harder for anyone to take the analysis seriously, and it leaves AHIP standing alone."[16]

I learned firsthand how outraged the White House was when I got a call from a senior White House official early on the morning that AHIP released the report. I was told that Ignagni herself had assured the White House just days before that AHIP had no plans to launch an immediate attack on the Baucus bill. It became clear to me during that conversation that the president and his aides had believed that industry leaders could be trusted. Now they understood why I had started speaking out against the industry and its duplicitous PR campaign, and they were hoping I would go after AHIP and its bogus study. I did, in my blog and in numerous interviews that week.

On October 13, the Finance Committee approved the Baucus bill 14–9, with a lone Republican "yes" vote cast by Senator Olympia Snowe of Maine. But AHIP's misstep did more than fail to kill reform—it briefly revived the fortunes of the public option. According to Shailagh Murray and Lori Montgomery of the *Washington Post*, Senate majority leader Harry Reid's "original inclination was to leave the public option out of a final bill he is writing from measures passed by the finance and health committees. But his liberal colleagues began urging him two weeks ago to reconsider, after insurance industry forecasts that premiums would rise sharply under the Finance Committee bill, which lacked a public option. The report had the effect of prodding Democrats to look for better ways to control costs, and the public option—strongly opposed by the insurance industry—reemerged as a possible solution."[17]

The impact of Reid including the public option in the merged

Senate bill was immediate. It ended Snowe's flirtation with bipartisan-ship. She announced that she would oppose the bill.

Meanwhile, Pelosi was trying to resolve differences among House Democrats. By adding stronger provisions barring illegal immigrants from buying insurance through government-run purchasing exchanges, even if they did not receive tax subsidies, and adding more restrictions on abortion coverage, Pelosi cobbled together the bare majority she needed to pass the bill. On November 7, the House voted 220–215 to pass the bill. One Republican, Joseph Cao of Louisiana, crossed party lines.

Now it was the Senate's turn, and the senior chamber worked twenty-five consecutive days, often debating into the night. Majority Leader Reid had to hold on to sixty votes to overcome a Republican filibuster, and he had fifty-eight Democrats plus two independents who caucused with them. One of them, Senator Joe Lieberman of Connecticut, said he would join a filibuster if the public option remained in the bill. Democrats proposed a trade that Lieberman had spoken favorably about earlier: allowing people aged fifty-five to sixty-four to buy into Medicare. But Lieberman commented that the idea must be bad if liberals favored it so strongly, and he nixed it as well, infuriating Democrats who howled about his hypocrisy. The other obstacle to sixty was Senator Ben Nelson (D-Neb.), a former insurance company CEO, who held out to the end—and was finally won over by a provision to funnel millions of dollars in extra Medicaid money to Nebraska. The deal was ridiculed as the "Cornhusker kickback" by Republicans and greeted with derision by Democrats, too, but they were happy just to see a deal. Now with his votes, Reid called the roll on Christmas Eve, and the bill was passed, 60–39. With the public option stripped from the bill, Lieberman joined the Democrats in voting for the bill. Senator Jim Bunning (R-Ky.) was the only member of the Senate who did not vote. The conference committee would take up the measure in January, and Congress emptied for the holidays.

Meanwhile, distracted by the Senate deliberations and the

holidays, a Democratic candidate expected to easily win a special election to replace Senator Kennedy (who had died on August 25) waged a
lackluster campaign. Massachusetts attorney general Martha Coakley
was so confident of winning that she took a New Year's vacation to the
Caribbean, did little polling, and bought minimal advertising. Her
GOP challenger, state senator Scott Brown, was traveling the state in
his pickup and firing up a conservative base that wanted nothing more
than to take the sixtieth vote in the Senate away from the Democrats in
the January 19 election. They got their wish: Brown trounced Coakley,
52 percent to 47 percent.

Obama and the stunned Democrats huddled to figure out whether
health care reform could be salvaged. The Tea Party, their Freedom-
Works enablers, and the insurance industry that funded them were
elated at the growing likelihood that they would kill reform and undercut Obama's presidency.

Pelosi and Reid took several weeks to devise a strategy to push
reform through both chambers despite the addition of Brown as the
forty-first vote against the bill. If the House could pass the Senate bill,
unchanged from Christmas Eve, there would be no need for a conference bill requiring sixty Senate votes. But Pelosi knew that some House
Democrats were unhappy with the Senate bill and would reject it unless they could count on a companion bill with House fixes that could
be adopted in the Senate with fifty-one votes under reconciliation.

As this plan took shape, Obama appeared in an interview on the
Super Bowl pre-game show and announced that he would lead another
White House "summit" that would be broadcast on national television.
Americans could watch as the two parties discussed how they might
make a deal on health care reform. Some argue that his true purpose
was to shine a light on the paucity of Republican ideas and their
unwillingness to work in good faith with the administration and congressional leaders.

Even with the president fully engaged, I could sense that Democrats in Congress were not confident they could pull off their plan.

Within days, however, they got an unexpected gift from the insurance industry. The *Los Angeles Times* reported in early February that California's largest health insurer, Anthem Blue Cross, a subsidiary of WellPoint, had notified eight hundred thousand of its customers that it was going to raise their premiums by as much as 39 percent.[18] The move sparked a backlash that attracted national media attention. Obama, Secretary Sebelius, and congressional Democrats seized on the planned rate increase and kept the story alive for days, overshadowing the Republicans' continuing efforts to kill "Obamacare," as they were calling the reform legislation.

In early March, Obama exhorted Democratic lawmakers to finish the bill by the Easter recess. Pelosi and Reid went ahead with the reconciliation plan over vitriolic GOP objections. The Republicans complained that the Democrats were using a procedural "nuclear option" to push the legislation through. Reid reminded them of all the major bills they had passed using the same procedure when they had controlled the Senate during the Bush administration—including two huge tax cuts and the creation of an industry-backed Medicare prescription drug program.

Pelosi and Reid had numerous other problems to resolve, not the least of which was opposition to the legislation from a group of Democrats who wanted to strengthen restrictions on abortions. There were also liberals who still hoped for a public option.

Obama warned both groups that the time had come to pass reform or the party would suffer in November. The final hurdle was leaped when the most ardent antiabortion Democrat in the House, Bart Stupak of Michigan, said he would vote for the bill if Obama signed an executive order reassuring him that language in the legislation could not be interpreted to offer women easy access to abortions.

On Sunday night, March 21, 2010, Pelosi banged the gavel and declared the Senate bill passed by a vote of 219–212. That action was followed immediately by the passage of a "sidecar" bill to change a few sections of the Senate bill that House Democrats didn't like. The *unless reconcilable.*

Senate would later pass the final bill, sending it to the president for
his signature.

And it was done.

The law is imperfect in many ways, but if it had not been enacted,
the chances of health care reform happening anytime soon would have
been remote. The insurance industry and other special interests would
have made sure of that.

As for me, I will never know if anything I did during the debate
made a difference in its outcome—but I can say without doubt that I
was more proud of what I had done over those several months than of
anything I had ever done in my long career as a PR executive.

Telling the truth is very cathartic. I highly recommend it.

CHAPTER XI

The Playbook

L ET'S say you are the CEO of a big corporation not held in especially high esteem by the public. Maybe your company sells health insurance, drills for oil in the Gulf of Mexico, makes billions of dollars from trading derivatives, or even makes food items craved by the masses—like soda or other sugary beverages.

Now let's pretend that things are not going well for you at the moment. Congress and the White House or local governments across the country are proposing new legislation or new taxes on your products that will force you to change the way you do business, operate in a more socially responsible way, or maybe even accept a lower profit margin.

The big investors who own most of the shares in your company will not be happy if any of these things happen. And you already know what they will do when they aren't happy: sell their shares by the millions, forcing your company's stock price down, and along with it the value of your own stock options. Because your top priority as CEO is to "enhance shareholder value," your job will be on the line if your board of directors concludes you're not up to the task.

So, what are you going to do to keep those bad things from happening? If you're like many other CEOs, you'll turn to "The Playbook on How to Influence Lawmakers and Regulators Through the Manipulation of Public Opinion."

Until now, this playbook has been so carefully guarded by the people who make millions of dollars for their corporate customers by using it, the non-CEO you probably didn't even know it existed. Another reason you've likely never heard of the playbook is that, like most people, you probably didn't even notice the manipulation was taking place.

The playbook—which I will share with you shortly—has evolved over the years as a result of advances in technology and changes in how people get their information. But in many ways, it is the same playbook that was developed decades ago for an industry that consistently inhabits the lowest realm of public esteem: the tobacco industry.

There is little doubt that the tobacco industry set the standard for manipulating public opinion and dodging regulation. No discussion of this topic can start without first considering the king of spin and manipulation: big tobacco. To get an idea of what our country—and the world—is up against in the way of corporate deception, you must understand this industry.

Despite the well-known lethal effects of their products, cigarette makers have managed to keep them firmly entrenched in society's mainstream. The industry's behind-the-scenes activities to accomplish this have been so vast, so clever, so highly financed, and so pervasive that it's impossible to list them all. We'll probably never know everything big tobacco did out of public view, but since that industry's maneuvers are so important to the history of spin and how it is carried out today, I need to briefly describe them.

Cigarettes are deadly when used as intended and kill over 443,000 Americans a year. Their makers engineer them for addiction, attractiveness, taste and "smoothness," and ease of use.[1] No other legal product has these dangerous characteristics, yet cigarettes are shockingly unregulated for the amount of carnage they produce.

Governments and public health groups have been struggling for decades to overcome the industry's efforts to confuse the public about the health hazards of smoking. The question is, how did this industry go about achieving its objectives, and what can we learn from its activities?

The tobacco industry is really two industries: One makes and sells cigarettes, and the other engages in a full-time effort to foster doubt about criticisms of tobacco products, encourage distrust of government, manipulate legislative processes, distract people from the negative effects, neutralize and harass opponents, coerce and coordinate allies, undermine scientific and common knowledge—and persuade people that smoking is normal, even helpful, human behavior.

WHAT THE INDUSTRY DID AND HOW IT DID IT

Perhaps the best way to demonstrate the scale of the tobacco industry's subversive behavior is to delve into some of its internal projects, beginning with one of the most recent. The Regulatory Strategy Project was a long-term Philip Morris (PM) effort to get Food and Drug Administration regulations passed that were in the company's favor. It took ten years to achieve that goal, but when Congress approved a new FDA tobacco bill and President Obama signed it into law in 2009, PM got what it had sought.

PM had started driving the creation of the FDA bill to regulate tobacco in 1999, and the company worked steadily behind the scenes to craft and engineer its passage. The bill adhered to a list of internal "core principles" that the company had outlined early in 2000, including the tenets that the FDA not be able to alter basic cigarette design or interfere with cigarette marketing. PM also wanted to keep its ingredients secret and keep the FDA from "infringing on the right of adult Americans to choose to take the risks of smoking."[2] In addition, the company wanted a bill that would prevent the FDA from removing nicotine from cigarettes entirely (so that addiction could be maintained). These protections and others were built into the final bill.

Longtime tobacco-control activists warned that PM was driving the legislation, not public health authorities. They warned that the bill would tie the hands of the FDA, turning it into a de facto research and development department for cigarette manufacturers—as well as giving PM a market advantage over its competitors, who also protested that the bill would help PM at their expense. Among other things, the bill exempted existing tobacco products, giving them "grandfathered" status, and was worded in such a way as to discourage the development of new tobacco products, even those that PM's competitors had been working on that might be considerably safer than the grandfathered cigarettes. Despite these red flags, Congress passed the bill, handing PM so many advantages that both rival tobacco companies and public health advocates dubbed it the "Marlboro Protection Act" (Marlboro being one of the brands manufactured by PM). Amid debate over the bill, Senator Mike Enzi (R-Wyo.), ranking member of the Senate Health, Education, Labor, and Pensions Committee, confirmed publicly on May 21, 2009, that PM—the tobacco company itself—had co-authored the bill.[3] So how did we get to this point?

SMOKERS HAVE RIGHTS, TOO, YOU KNOW

Earlier, in the 1970s and 1980s, the industry had realized that it lacked a counterpart to grassroots antismoking efforts being organized by groups like the American Lung Association, the American Heart Association, and the American Cancer Society. No one was jumping to the industry's defense as these groups taught people about the dangers of smoking, helped smokers quit, and lobbied for smoke-free public places.

To remedy this inequity, PM and R. J. Reynolds (RJR) quietly organized "smokers' rights groups" throughout the country. They were managed by PR firms that activated them to rise to the industry's defense on local issues like tobacco taxes and smoking bans. The industry wanted the groups to seem like spontaneous uprisings of angry, beleaguered, suppressed smokers, and the PR firms that ran them shielded cigarette makers from being detected as the creators. By July 1994, the American tobacco industry had spent about ten million dollars and recruited around three hundred thousand members into these groups, with a goal of one million by the end of that year.[4]

(Taking a page from that playbook, AHIP in 1999 created the ongoing fake grassroots campaign Coalition for Medicare Choices to get senior citizens who were enrolled in private insurers' Medicare Advantage plans to do the industry's PR and lobbying work. The federal government has been overpaying insurers more than twelve billion dollars a year to offer these plans to seniors. The overpayments have made significant contributions to the bottom lines of most of the big insurers, especially Humana and UnitedHealth, which is why the industry has spent millions every year in PR and lobbying efforts to keep the program from being eliminated. AHIP's member companies and their PR firms have recruited an estimated four hundred thousand seniors, who participate in town hall meetings and contact members of Congress through phone calls, e-mails, and letters. AHIP has also used millions of policyholders' premium dollars to fly thousands of Medicare Advantage enrollees to Washington to lobby for the insurers whenever Congress has threatened to reduce the overpayments.)

RJR called its original effort to create smokers' rights groups the Partisan Project. The company had spent years accumulating personal information on smokers, and it used this massive database to contact smokers and help them "develop an affinity with other [individual smokers]." RJR sought to "create awareness of discriminatory situations" that presented "avenues for opposition" for smokers to protest smoking bans. The Partisan Project was aimed at "instilling and reinforcing feelings of effectiveness" in smokers, and creating the appearance that massive numbers of smokers were spontaneously speaking out to oppose public health measures.

As part of the project, RJR pressed its sales force to serve as an "alert network on local anti-smoking issues." Once the Partisan program was in place, the company used "a public relations program [to communicate] to the general public that opposition to smoker discrimination is growing."[5] RJR test-marketed the Partisan Project in Colorado, Texas, and Florida, where the company hired state and local field coordinators to head up groups, establishing toll-free telephone numbers and urging smokers to provide it with names of other smokers who might be interested in joining.

PM formed a similar group in the early 1990s called the National Smokers Alliance, which portrayed smokers as targets of prejudice and tried to motivate them to "fight back." Also to give the appearance of grassroots opposition and hide the company's involvement, PM used the NSA to fight the 1993 Clinton health care reform plan, which would have been paid for in part by a cigarette tax. PM hired the big PR firm Burson-Marsteller to operate the NSA, with the goal of targeting fifty million smokers to "rile up and mobilize a committed cadre of hundreds of thousands, better yet millions, to be foot soldiers in a grassroots army directed by Philip Morris' political operatives at Burson-Marsteller."[6] The NSA also promoted PM's Accommodation Program—a project to preserve smoking in restaurants and bars.

OUR PRODUCTS KILL, BUT WE'RE SOCIALLY RESPONSIBLE

In an attempt to improve the industry's image, tobacco companies have also touted their "corporate social responsibility" activities, one of the most prominent of which was the industry's "youth smoking prevention" program.

In 1991, RJR characterized the youth-smoking issue as "the most potent weapon that anti-smokers can bring to bear against the tobacco industry."[7] In response to pressure over the issue, the industry introduced a string of "youth access" programs with names like It's the Law, We Card, and Action Against Access—all nominally aimed at preventing cigarette sales to youth. Suddenly, "We Card" stickers and placards started turning up at the entrances of convenience stores all across the country. This U-turn—from wanting kids to smoke to saying they didn't want kids to smoke—was hard for many people to swallow. It generated skepticism about these programs, and rightly so. What the programs *really* did was much worse than merely being disingenuous. The programs had highly damaging applications.

Around the time that big tobacco introduced its first youth-access programs, antitobacco advocates had given up trying to beat the industry at the state and federal levels. These higher levels of government were too tightly controlled by the industry and were no longer very responsive to activists. So antitobacco proponents had begun approaching their city council members, who were more responsive and less likely to be swayed by corporate influence. Smoking bans had started appearing in local jurisdictions around the country, and progress had been made in getting smoking out of restaurants and workplaces.

Alarmed by the shift, the tobacco industry realized it was vulnerable. Because it had no similar national grassroots networks to oppose these local efforts, it started retailer programs like We Card to defeat them.

Youth programs served the industry on several levels. They gave it cover against the charge that it targeted kids, and they generated goodwill among legislators. But these retailer programs also served another function: They gave the industry an opening to have company representatives conduct personal visits with retailers all over the country. Under the guise of instructing retailers to check for IDs as part of a youth-access program, industry representatives also asked retailers to monitor political activity in their towns—and paid them to report back to the Tobacco Institute, the industry's former trade and lobbying group, at the first appearance of any problems (like citizens pushing for a smoking ban), so the institute could mobilize.

An institute document made public years later stated, "For monitoring purposes, we fund our allies in the convenience store groups to regularly report on ordinance introductions and assist in campaigns to stop unreasonable measures . . . Promotion of The Institute's 'It's the Law' program and other industry programs play a helpful role." It added that "the bottom line is that if we do not know a local battle is taking place in a timely manner, there is no way in which we can employ our resources to challenge unfair outcomes."[8]

Retailers as well as restaurant and bar owners across the country started phoning the Tobacco Institute to let it know about "trouble" in their area, and the industry responded by flying representatives to those towns to generate and coordinate strident opposition—or at least the appearance of strident opposition—to the antismoking efforts.

No corner of the country, no jerkwater town, was too small for the industry's attempts at intervention. It knew that once people experienced smoke-free places, the trend would spread. So it sent people, often smokers'-rights-group organizers, to the smallest, most remote little towns to squelch these activities as soon as they got started.

In addition to using youth programs to help fight smoking bans, the industry used them to help fight cigarette taxes and marketing restrictions. The programs also generated goodwill with the governments of some foreign countries and even allowed PM to partner with foreign health ministries. In 2001, the company announced that it was "actively involved in more than 130 [youth-smoking prevention] programs in more than 70 countries." The idea was to make people around the world think that tobacco companies were straightening themselves out before lawmakers could do it for them.

SOCIAL ENGINEERING

It is widely known that the tobacco industry hired scientists to spin its messages about the health effects of tobacco and secondhand smoke, but beyond manipulating hard science by commissioning the creation of positive scientific studies and infusing them into the press and other media, the industry also recruited a wide range of "soft scientists"—sociologists, philosophers, political scientists, psychologists, and economists—to influence public opinion through cultural routes.

For example, the industry recruited economists who produced "studies" based on nonscientific, anecdotal evidence that "showed" that smoking bans hurt business. The industry disseminated these studies through credible third parties and used them to scare restaurant, bar, and hotel owners into helping fight smoking bans, by generating fear over the bans' financial consequences.

It worked for decades. Whenever the public pushed for a law restricting smoking in restaurants, restaurant owners would claim they were afraid of losing business and point to "reports" secretly generated by the tobacco industry that predicted economic doom if smoking bans were passed.

The industry also paid professional philosophers to come up with new arguments in favor of tobacco that did not touch on the subject of health. On February 1, 2002, the U.K. *Guardian* exposed prominent British philosophy professor Roger Scruton, who the newspaper said was secretly taking payments from Japan Tobacco to write pro-smoking articles and place them in a slew of prestigious newspapers and international magazines.[9] Scruton wrote articles deriding public health advocacy and warning about the forthcoming "nanny state"—a phrase politicians still use regularly.

Scruton helped the tobacco industry spread skepticism about government-led public safety efforts. In a 1998 article titled "A Snort of Derision at Society," Scruton claimed that seat belt laws caused people to drive faster, thus nullifying any apparent boost in safety that the law created.[10] In another article, he extolled "the benefits of risk taking" and argued that smoking was healthy for its stress-relieving benefits.

Big insurance is grateful to big tobacco not only for its groundbreaking work in stealth PR but also because the tobacco industry consistently ranks lower—although just slightly—than the health insurance industry in terms of public trust and esteem. And when the public doesn't think your company or industry can be trusted to tell the truth or do the right thing, you have to recruit third parties and create front groups to do the communicating for you. PM turned some of the first shovels of dirt in these deceptive techniques to manipulate opinion.

To get around its lack of credibility and to hide its hand in influencing public beliefs, PM created additional front groups. The company hired PR firms to create artificial third-party organizations and assign each one a cause, like counteracting government health warnings about its industry's products. This allowed the company to create entirely separate, far more credible mouthpieces to advance its political ends.

In 1993, at PM's instigation, multinational tobacco companies created a European social engineering front group called Associates for Research into the Science of Enjoyment (ARISE). PM was ARISE's primary funder, but the group got additional financing from RJR, Rothmans, and British American Tobacco in the United Kingdom—as well as from the companies' respective food and drink subsidiaries, like Kraft, Miller Beer, and Nestlé. The tobacco companies created ARISE to counteract a U.S. surgeon general's report that compared nicotine addiction to heroin and cocaine addiction.

This likening of nicotine to heroin and cocaine sent up red flags throughout the global tobacco industry. The answer—without letting the public know that the industry was behind it—was ARISE, whose job was essentially to undermine government efforts to warn people about the highly addictive characteristic of nicotine. Of course, as with other front groups, the management of ARISE was farmed out to a PR firm, Fishburn Hedges, in the United Kingdom.[11]

ARISE's "expert" members were portrayed—through press releases, articles, interviews, and media tours—as impartial academic and scientific authorities who felt compelled to address the "science of pleasure." They held conferences, published books, toured continents, generated media events and newspaper and magazine articles, created video news releases and press releases, and wrote letters to the editor, all while keeping secret the fact that the group's activities were backed by the tobacco industry.

PROMOTING THE IDEA OF "JUNK SCIENCE"

After the Environmental Protection Agency declared secondhand smoke a Class A human carcinogen in 1993, PM once again desperately needed a powerful "group" to rise up, this time to help discredit the EPA's findings. So it created The Advancement of Sound Science Coalition (TASSC).

PM looked around for help funding such a group, and the chemical, paper, metal, petroleum, and other environmentally dubious industries were thrilled to help a group of "committed experts" who would say publicly that scientific warnings against *their* activities were a bunch of baloney, too. So, with other willing industries waiting with wallets open, PM created TASSC—working, as with all its other groups, through a PR firm later favored by the health insurance industry, APCO Worldwide. After a feasibility study conducted with PM's law firm, Covington and Burling, APCO began the campaign.

APCO did an admirable job of recruiting members for TASSC. The "supporters list" included everything from down-home-sounding businesses like the Family Loompya Seafood Market and Pinckneyville Lighting to sawmills and mining and chemical companies (including W. R. Grace, Amoco, and Dow Chemical). TASSC was assigned three basic talking points: (1) Science should never be corrupted to achieve political ends; (2) economic growth cannot afford to be held hostage to paternalistic overregulation; and (3) improving indoor air quality is a laudable goal that will never be accomplished as long as tobacco smoke is the sole focus of regulators.[12]

TASSC worked to hang the label of "junk science" on warnings that secondhand smoke caused health problems for nonsmokers. Eventually, the group hung the same junk-science label on environmentalists, and it went on to advance industry-friendly positions on a wide range of topics, including global warming, phthalates, and pesticides. Diversifying this way helped PM continue obtaining other industries' help with funding the group, and with further disguising the group's tobacco origins.[13]

THE PLAYBOOK FUNDAMENTALS

The tobacco industry's PR strategies have been so broad based, well funded, and stunningly successful that other industries—not just health insurers—are adopting them rapid-fire. The tobacco industry has, in effect, injected its negative, manipulating DNA into corporate culture worldwide, to the detriment of people everywhere.

To emulate that industry's success, here are actions that you, as an embattled CEO (or your trade association), must take:

• Hire a big and well-connected PR firm, preferably one that has established a reputation not so much for public "relations" as for public "deception." The firm should pay little or no attention to the Public Relations Society of America's Code of Ethics, which, among other things, insists that PR practitioners disclose who they are working for and refrain from engaging in deceit. Fortunately, many of the biggest firms pay little heed to such ethical guidelines. They are more than happy to take your money to:
• Set up and operate a coalition or front group, which, if at all possible, should have words like "American" or "freedom" or "choice" in its name. You can launder your money through your PR firm so that no one has to know you have any association with the front group. The PR firm will also:
• Recruit third parties to list as members of your front group. Depending on the scope of your problems and the issues you

are battling, the members can range from mom-and-pop bodega owners and motel operators to the U.S. Chamber of Commerce and the National Federation of Independent Business, both of which, by the way, have long track records of lending their names to stealth campaigns. Your PR firm will also maximize the effectiveness of your third parties by helping them:

• Write letters to the editor and op-eds and place them in local and national publications. In fact, the PR firm will do all the writing and placing. The third parties won't have to do a thing except lend their names. The letters and op-eds will convey all the key messages that you yourself would convey but cannot because doing so would be perceived, correctly, as self-serving. To be sure those letters and op-eds get published in the right places, your PR firm must:

• Cultivate close relationships with editors and publishers. Chances are, your firm will have PR pros on staff who once worked at the publications and other news outlets important to you and your industry. Because of their relationships with key reporters, those PR people will also be able to:

• Influence the tone and content of articles that those reporters write about your company and your industry. This is especially important if you are in the midst of a well-publicized crisis. To bolster your point of view and give reporters an all-important angle, your PR firm might need to:

• Conduct a bogus survey or slice and dice data with the intent of misleading, or "lying with statistics." And your firm's PR pros will also know how to:

• Feed talking points to TV pundits and frequent contributors to op-ed pages. They will know how to get talk show hosts with big audiences like Rush Limbaugh or Bill O'Reilly or Glenn Beck to say things on the air to support your point of view and discredit your opponents. Lastly, using varying tactics that will depend on the nature of your problem, your PR firm will:

• Develop and carry out a duplicitous communications campaign. Whenever you need to comment publicly, your firm will
help you make sure that what you say is perceived to be positive,
that you are seen as being responsible and cooperative, and that
the public and lawmakers feel that they can count on you to do the
right thing and be honest and straightforward. This is the charm
offensive I've talked about. To distract from the fact that your
product is widely considered to be a problem, your PR firm will
develop a creative campaign to position your company or
industry as part of the solution. It will also broaden the issue to
take attention off your maligned product, and it will stress how
many people your company employs and how much it contrib-
utes to the local or national economy. Behind the scenes, your
firm will be using the front groups and their devious tactics to
do the necessary dirty work for you.

These are the fundamental tools of the spin business. There are
many others, of course, but these are tried-and-true and have worked
for big corporations and their trade groups for decades. Following are
some "ripped from the headlines" examples of how they are being deployed today by three big industries.

BIG OIL

When an offshore drilling rig exploded in the Gulf of Mexico on April
20, 2010, killing eleven people and creating a massive oil spill, BP
launched a multipronged PR strategy as soon as it had begun efforts
to try to cap the gusher, which threatened miles of U.S. coastline.

In an attempt to persuade Americans, especially those living and
vacationing along the Gulf Coast, that it was a socially responsible company doing all it could do to contain the mess it had made, BP enlisted
the support of local businesses and state tourism agencies to allay concerns that the region's beaches and flora and fauna were threatened.

The Daily Beast Web site reported on May 19, 2010, that BP had quietly shelled out more than seventy million dollars to produce and air commercials ostensibly meant to lure tourists to the area but subliminally implying that BP had done what local businesses and governments had expected it to do in cleaning up the oil spill.[14]

"It's one piece of an enormous, largely stealth PR campaign that BP has been waging over the past few weeks . . . as the enormity of the Deepwater Horizon rig disaster sinks in," Daily Beast reporter Rick Outzen wrote. He added that "the ground operatives in this propaganda blitz are locally-owned or affiliated companies—mostly those that either supply or own BP stations."

"Specifically," he continued, citing sources inside the oil industry, "while BP has commandeered the state's tourism marketing, the oil giant wants its local marketers to buy ads, distribute flyers at their stations, hold customer appreciation days and use BP-supplied talking points to build a word-of-mouth campaign to 'diffuse or deflect negative commentary' about the BP oil spill." BP had pledged to cover all their expenses.

Originally known as British Petroleum, the company changed its name to BP in 2000 "to project a more environmentally friendly image, saying the initials stood for 'Beyond Petroleum,'" *Newsweek* noted in a May 17, 2010, article about how before the catastrophe in the Gulf the company had vigorously fought additional federal regulation of oil drilling in coastal waters.[15] The article quoted Dave Levinthal of the Center for Responsive Politics as saying that BP had in recent years—which coincided with the company's multi-million-dollar campaign to reinforce its image as a "green" company—increased its lobbying in Washington "exponentially" to dilute new laws on the prevention of oil-spill pollution.

Thus, on the one hand it had been quietly lobbying Congress to loosen environmental-protection laws, while on the other it had been promoting itself publicly as environmentally friendly. By most accounts, the company's ongoing campaign to paint itself green was a big success. "BP is running a greenwashing campaign, and from a sales and marketing perspective, it is brilliant," said John Stauber of the Center for Media and Democracy (CMD) in the January 14, 2008, edition of *Adweek*.[16]

Big oil companies have worked closely with other energy and fossil fuel industries—coal companies in particular—to persuade Americans that climate change not only is nothing to worry about but also is not even happening. The modus operandi of these industries—and the front groups that they have their PR firms create and run—is to create fear that efforts to address a problem that they contend doesn't really exist will hurt the economy and cost jobs.

One of the leaders in the campaign to diminish concerns about the role that coal-fired power plants play in climate change is the American Coalition for Clean Coal Electricity (previously known as the Center for Energy and Economic Development, or CEED). A leaked 2004 memo from the organization, obtained in 2009 by the CMD, described how it was working behind the scenes to keep both the legislative and the judicial branches of government from taking any actions on climate change that would affect the industry in a negative way.

"In the climate change arena," the memo stated, "CEED focuses on three areas: opposing government-mandated controls of greenhouse gases (GHG), opposing 'regulation by litigation,' and supporting sequestration technology as the proper vehicles for addressing any reasonable concerns about greenhouse gas concentrations in the atmosphere."

The CMD also discovered that CEED's PR firm was the Hawthorn Group, a Virginia-based firm that the health insurance industry has hired to fight anti-managed-care legislation and litigation. (I participated in numerous strategy-development sessions with Hawthorn Group staffers and my counterparts from other big insurers after several class action lawsuits were filed against our employers on behalf of physicians and their patients in 2000.)

The Hawthorn Group crowed about its successes on behalf of

CEED in a 2008 newsletter it sent to "friends and family." Two paragraphs are particularly noteworthy:

> The program also had an impact on the perception of coal among public opinion leaders. In September 2007, on the key measurement question—Do you support/oppose the use of coal to generate electricity?—we found 46 percent support and 50 percent oppose. In a 2008 year-end survey that result had shifted to 72 percent support and 22 percent oppose. Not only did we see significantly increased support, opposition was cut by more than half. Republican presidential candidate Sen. John McCain addressed a crowd wearing "Clean Coal hats" in Pennsylvania.
>
> Building on our existing 200,000-strong grassroots citizen army, we leveraged the presidential candidates' own supporters, finding advocates for clean coal among the crowd to carry our message. We got these on-the-spot advocates to show strong public support to the candidates and to the media, and enhanced that visibility by integrating online media that created even more of a buzz. We did this by sending "clean coal" branded teams to hundreds of presidential candidate events, carrying a positive message (we can be part of the solution to climate change) which was reinforced by giving away free T-shirts and hats emblazoned with our branding: Clean Coal. Attendees at the candidate events wore these items into the events.[*]

Another front group funded by oil companies, the American Energy Alliance, began running ads in late 2009 warning that American taxpayers would pay a heavy price if legislation designed to slow global warming were approved. The AEA was formed in 1993 by the American Petroleum Institute and several large corporations to defeat a bill that would have made companies polluting the environment pay for their emissions.

---

[*] Beware of anyone or any group that claims to be "part of the solution." Trust me.

The AEA ads claimed that the bill would cost families more than three thousand dollars a year in new taxes. Headed by a former staff member of Tom DeLay (the former Republican House majority leader), the AEA got that number from a Massachusetts Institute of Technology study estimating that the bill would cost roughly that amount per taxpayer. What the AEA did not disclose was that the MIT study said that taxpayers would not pay any of it.[17] The author of the study, John Reilly, said that the claims made by the AEA and its allies in Congress were false.

In addition, the Web site NaturalNews noted, "The AEA ads fail to mention the bill's emphasis on increased energy efficiency, which would actually save consumers and businesses money—an estimated $465 billion per year, according to a Union of Concerned Scientists study. If the government uses money raised by the bill to finance tax breaks or other incentives for consumers to retrofit their homes for more efficiency, the average household would save $900, including $580 on fuel and $320 on electricity, heating and cooking."

One of the world's leading experts on climate change, Joseph Romm, told the online magazine Guernica that the campaigns on behalf of the industry to manipulate public opinion have been stunningly successful. "The fossil-fuel companies and the right-wing have been very effective in their disinformation campaign," said Romm, a physicist and founder of the Center for Energy and Climate Solutions, whom *Time* magazine named one of its Heroes for the Environment in 2009. "It's the most successful disinformation campaign in human history." As a result, he said, even progressive politicians "have been persuaded not to talk so much about global warming."[18]

BIG SODA

With evidence mounting that sugary sodas and other beverages are a leading contributor to the obesity epidemic in the United States, Congress, some states, and several American cities have considered imposing a special tax on the drinks to reduce consumption and also generate needed revenue to help pay for municipal services. In early 2010, Philadelphia mayor Michael Nutter proposed a two-cents-per-ounce tax on all sweetened drinks, and in Washington, D.C., city council member Mary Cheh proposed a one-cent-per-ounce tax on bottled and canned soda that contained sugar.

Alarmed, the beverage industry sprang into action to defeat efforts to impose a special tax of any amount on its products. Among the first things the industry did was hire a big PR firm to set up a front group, Americans Against Food Taxes. Funded primarily by beverage and food companies and their lobbying groups, AAFT was formed initially to fight a proposed three- to ten-cent tax on sodas and other sugary drinks that health care reform advocates in Congress had proposed to help pay for the expansion of insurance coverage in the new health care bill.

To obscure its real source of funding, AAFT describes itself as a "coalition of concerned citizens—responsible individuals, financially strapped families, small and large businesses in communities across the country" opposed to any government-proposed tax on sugar-sweetened drinks. But as disclosed on the CMD's SourceWatch Web site, the group's membership consists mainly of lobbying groups for packaged-food and soda companies, chain restaurant corporations, and large food and soft drink manufacturers and distributors—including the Coca-Cola Company, Dr Pepper–Royal Crown Bottling Company, PepsiCo, Canada Dry Bottling Company of New York, the Can Manufacturers Institute, 7-Eleven Convenience Stores, and Yum! Brands.

The CMD's investigation found that the group's Web site, www .nofoodtaxes.com, is registered to Goddard Claussen, the PR and advertising firm that conjured up the "Harry and Louise" commercials to help defeat the Clinton health care reform plan.

Using the "we're part of the solution" tactic, AAFT launched a campaign to persuade Americans that beverage companies are doing their part to get kids to cut down on their consumption of high-calorie sodas. The group has used ads and e-mail blasts to boast that soda companies have replaced full-calorie soft drinks with "smaller-portion" and "portion controlled" beverages, real juice, and bottled water. Voilà! Their products are no longer the problem; they are part of the solution. Even better, now they will get kids to buy more bottled water—which costs the companies next to nothing to make—at a dollar a bottle, more than they would pay for a soda.

Another part of AAFT's campaign is to generate outrage against a soda tax by calling it a tax on "groceries." It isn't a tax on groceries; it's just a tax on one class of foods: sugary drinks. But by shifting the focus, the group stands a better chance of getting people—especially low-income people—to oppose the tax.

To kill Nutter's proposal in Philadelphia, the Pennsylvania Beverage Association created a coalition with local businesses—including owners of bodegas throughout the city—and even a labor union, the Teamsters, because its members delivered sodas to stores, restaurants, and schools. The coalition conducted a fearmongering campaign, arguing that the tax would ruin small-business owners and lead to layoffs in the beverage and transportation industries.

In the weeks leading up to the Philadelphia City Council's vote on the proposed beverage tax, the beverage industry mounted a full-court press, including sending the spokesman for the American Beverage Association to the city "to plot strategy," according to the *Philadelphia Inquirer.* "Lobbyists are buttonholing City Council members," the *Inquirer* reported. "Trade groups and the unions have locked arms. Industry ads are sprouting on the air and in print extolling the good corporate citizenship of soft-drink companies. The public has weighed in with hundreds of calls and e-mails."[19]

The strategy worked. In May 2010, despite being millions of dollars short in paying for city services, council members voted down the tax but approved a budget with a projected $130 million shortfall. To help close the budget gap, the council voted to raise property taxes by almost 10 percent, but Nutter said even that wouldn't raise enough revenue to avoid cutbacks. He also said, after the defeat of his proposal, that the city would have to cut police, fire, and library services and eliminate 339 jobs.

Nutter blamed the beverage industry's intense PR and lobbying campaign for the demise of the proposed soda tax and the need to lay off city workers. "They will literally attempt to do or say anything to prevent what is essentially a good idea," he told the *Philadelphia Daily News*.[20]

The beverage industry's win in Philadelphia was just the latest in its string of victories. The proposed tax in Washington succumbed the same week. Baltimore mayor Stephanie Rawlings-Blake saw her proposed tax stall in city council. The only place the industry did not prevail was Washington State, which approved an excise tax on soda, but as of this writing lobbyists were trying to persuade legislators to repeal it.

In Washington, D.C., Councilwoman Cheh summed up the situation well in a *Washington Post* story before the vote: "It's hard to fight a multimillion dollar PR effort from big soda."[21]

Indeed. The same article quoted Ellen Valentino, executive vice president of the Maryland-Delaware-D.C. Beverage Association, as saying that her group was prepared to spend "whatever it takes" to defeat the tax.

BIG BANKS

One of the PR tactics the banking industry used to defeat or water down financial reform legislation in 2010 was to try to fool Americans—especially liberals—into thinking that the legislation was another Wall Street bailout.

As the site Talking Points Memo (TPM) reported in April 2010, banks and their allies formed a front group they named Stop Too Big to Fail to carry out a massive disinformation campaign.

This front group—created by the same people who had launched a similar sham organization, funded by big telecom companies, to support deregulation of the cable industry—"entered the financial reform fray with $1.6 million in aid, a respected economist on board, a blitz of opinion columns on left-leaning websites, and a message cooked right into the group's name—Stop Too Big To Fail—that liberals could love," TPM reporter Justin Elliott wrote.[22]

"These guys make the KGB look like amateurs, and I used to work in Russia quite a lot," Simon Johnson, a prominent advocate of breaking up the big banks and a former chief economist at the International Monetary Fund, told TPM.

A central element of the group's strategy involved posting comments on the Huffington Post and launching diaries on liberal netroots sites like Daily Kos and FireDogLake. In its posts, the group paid "lip service to the idea of breaking up the big banks while at the same time adopting 'bailout fund' rhetoric used by Republicans, all the while devoting its resources to trying to kill financial reform altogether," according to TPM.

The group also reportedly had ties to DCI Group, which has set up numerous astroturf campaigns on behalf of big corporate clients, including the health insurance industry.

The group's ads ran in states represented by influential Democratic senators, including Majority Leader Harry Reid of Nevada, Claire McCaskill of Missouri, and Mark Warner of Virginia. They encouraged viewers to contact their senators and ask them to "vote against this phony financial reform and support real reform—stop 'too big to fail.'"

The truth was that the legislation contained explicit language designed to ensure that there would be no more bailouts of troubled banks, regardless of their size. It also gave additional powers to regulators to seize failing banks and break them up if necessary.

Goldman Sachs used another tried-and-true tactic to try to kill parts of the reform legislation it didn't like: saying one thing and working behind the scenes to do just the opposite. Goldman executives said in public statements that they supported the legislation, but, according to the Huffington Post Investigative Fund, they deployed an army of lobbyists on Capitol Hill to kill an important provision that would have prohibited banks from trading derivatives, which would have cost Goldman billions of dollars in revenue.[23]

Derivatives protect companies from the risks of investing in stocks, commodities, and mortgage-related securities. As the Huffington Post reported, Goldman and other banks sold risky mortgage-related securities to investors, using derivatives to bet that the securities would fail and profiting when they did. Such practices contributed to the 2008 global financial meltdown. Goldman was particularly concerned about the provision in the reform bill pertaining to derivatives because, according to Senate records, it could lose more than 40 percent of its profits if the regulations passed.

Goldman didn't get everything it wanted, despite the millions of dollars it spent on lobbying, but the final bill, which Congress passed in July 2010, and which contained several consumer protections, was still not comprehensive enough to keep banks from engaging in risky behavior.

All of the tactics used by the oil, beverage, and banking industries to influence lawmakers at every level of government were pulled straight from the cigarette makers' playbook: Distract people from the real problem; generate fear; split communities with rhetoric, pitting one group against another; encourage people to doubt scientific conclusions; question whether there really is a problem; and say one thing in public while working secretly to do the opposite.

This, regrettably, has become common practice in the corporate world.

If there is one message—and one that is actually true—it is this: Always look *behind* any public argument to see how your emotions are being manipulated.

And count on it. They are.

CHAPTER XII

Spinning Out of Control

THE nation's founding fathers so well understood the need for an informed public in their new democracy that they forbade Congress from restricting freedom of the press in the First Amendment to the Constitution, right along with guaranteeing freedom of speech and religion and the right to peaceably assemble.

In the 220 years since the ratification of the First Amendment, our mass communications have become more accessible, far reaching, and up-to-the-minute than ever, yet the need for reliable, objective information is as great as at any point in our history.

Today, we have arrived at a precarious moment. The number of credible news organizations, particularly newspapers, is declining. At the same time, the number of people, the amount of power, and the level of funding behind public relations efforts are greater than ever, and increasing. Americans are confronted daily—even hourly—with the daunting and growing challenge of deciphering truth from spin.

Alex Jones, director of Harvard University's Shorenstein Center on Press, Politics, and Public Policy, contends that American journalism is under assault. A former *New York Times* reporter and a Pulitzer Prize winner, Jones believes that the primary culprit is the same fuel that drives every other enterprise in the country: money. With the number of traditional news outlets on the decline, primarily because of dwindling circulation and advertising revenue, Jones has deep concerns that news may someday become available only to those who are willing and able to pay for it. Spin, of course, will remain freely available, and hard to miss.

This concept is disturbingly similar to that of health care being accessible only to those with the resources to pay what the market demands. "We may be headed for a world in which there is as yawning a disparity in accurate knowledge as there is in wealth," Jones wrote in 2009's *Losing the News*. "The elite will be deeply informed, and there will be a huge difference between what they know and what most other Americans know. We could be heading for a well-informed class at the top and a broad populace awash in opinion, spin, and propaganda."[1]

Jones's perspective on the price of news is reinforced by Rupert Murdoch, whose massive American media holdings include the Fox Broadcasting Company and the *Wall Street Journal*. Murdoch said in April 2010 that he believes print newspapers will survive . . . in electronic, pay-as-you-go formats. In an interview with Marvin Kalb on the TV program *The Kalb Report* Murdoch predicted that—despite polls to the contrary—people would be willing to pay for online news. "I think if people have no place else to go, they will pay for it—if it's not too much money."

As an example, Murdoch noted that users of the iPad, introduced in March 2010, were able to subscribe to the *WSJ* for only $4 a week. (He failed to point out that the iPad itself cost a minimum of $499, plus the additional cost of an Internet connection.) Murdoch insisted that news organizations should restrict access to their online information and said that the *WSJ* will "stop Google and Microsoft from taking our stories for nothing"—even when the information is credited and a link to the original story is provided. "Let them do their own reporting," he said.[2]

UNTIMELY DEATHS

A half a century ago—in the 1950s and '60s—most major American cities, and many minor ones, had at least two daily newspapers, and several had even more. There were both morning and afternoon papers, some of which shared the same printing presses, to report the news at the beginning of the day and at the end. As the pace of the news cycle increased and the influence of television grew, afternoon papers gradually shifted to a morning schedule or folded altogether, leaving late-day updates to the broadcast media. That simple formula for reporting the news of the day is long gone.

On February 26, 2009, the CEO of E. W. Scripps newspapers told the assembled staff of the 150-year-old *Rocky Mountain News*, one of Denver's two daily newspapers, that the paper would shut down after its regular editions the following day. "The industry is in serious, serious trouble," said Rich Boehne, explaining what the group already knew: that the paper had lost sixteen million dollars the year before and that Scripps had been unable to find a buyer since putting the *Rocky* on the block two months earlier.[3]

The demise of a well-respected daily newspaper in Denver was big news, but not because it was an unusual event. Quite the contrary: It was significant because it was part of the larger trend. The week before Boehne told the staff of the *Rocky*, which had won four Pulitzer Prizes in the previous decade, that the paper was "a victim of changing times in our industry and huge economic challenges," Hearst Newspapers announced that it was planning to close the *Seattle Post-Intelligencer* and was considering either closing or selling the *San Francisco Chronicle*.

A year later, the *Chronicle* was still the largest newspaper in northern California, but the *Post-Intelligencer* existed only in an on-line format. In the wake of the *Rocky*'s demise, some of its former staffers founded INDenverTimes (www.indenvertimes.com), an on-line publication dedicated to carrying on the journalistic mission of the deceased paper—but the venture was still scrambling for support and subscribers in spring 2010; indeed, a large percentage of Denver residents were unaware of the site's existence.

THE IRON CORE: NEWSPAPERS

Harvard's Jones describes news as a multilayered sphere. At the center is an "iron core of information" with a vast majority of it coming from traditional news organizations. Information in the "core" encompasses fact-based local, national, and international news—which Jones calls "accountability news" because its purpose is to hold accountable those people in power, in both government and business, whose decisions and actions drive events. "Traditional journalists," Jones wrote in *Losing the News*, "have long believed that this form of fact-based accountability news is the essential food supply of democracy, and that without enough of this healthy nourishment, democracy will weaken, sicken, or even fail."[4]

In Jones's news sphere, this iron core is surrounded by a thick layer of talk and opinion, which derives from the core news. In other words, advocacy information—every talk show, radio commentary, crowd-rousing speech, and letter to the editor—depends on a basic core of information provided by objective news reporting. Jones contends that the decline of core reporting means that commentary has drifted further and further from factual news. "There will be a bounty of talk—the news of assertion—but serious news, reported by professional journalists, is running scared," he wrote in *Losing the News*, adding,

> The biggest worry of those concerned about the news is that this iron core is in jeopardy, largely because of the troubles plaguing the newspaper business. It is the nation's newspapers that provide the vast majority of iron core news. My own estimate is that 85 percent of professionally reported accountability news comes from

newspapers, but I have heard guesses from credible sources that go as high as 95 percent. While people may *think* they get their news from television or the Web, when it comes to this kind of news, it is almost always newspapers that have done the actual reporting.[5]

With circulations dropping, traditional newspaper advertisers are turning elsewhere to reach potential customers, which means less ad revenue to pay for reporters' salaries and the high cost of producing and distributing printed news. (Unlike the *Wall Street Journal*, which has a fairly stable circulation and plenty of well-to-do readers who are willing to pay for online content, most daily newspapers have found that their readers will go elsewhere for information if the papers try to charge for their stories on the Web.) Government reports show that the number of newspaper jobs in the United States began declining in the late 1990s—more than one hundred thousand were lost in the ensuing decade. According to U.S. census data, employment in the newspaper-publishing industry dropped by 25.4 percent in the eight years between 2001 and 2009.[6]

"The Reconstruction of American Journalism," a report published in the *Columbia Journalism Review (CJR)* in October 2009, stated, "Newspapers and television news are not going to vanish in the foreseeable future, despite frequent predictions of their imminent extinction. But they will play diminished roles in an emerging and still rapidly changing world of digital journalism, in which the means of news reporting are being re-invented, the character of news is being reconstructed, and reporting is being distributed across a greater number and variety of news organizations, new and old."

The *CJR* report explained the risks of the current trend: "What is under threat is independent *reporting* that provides information, investigation, analysis, and community knowledge, particularly in the coverage of local affairs . . . It may not be essential to save any particular news medium, including printed newspapers. What is paramount is preserving independent, original, credible reporting, whether or not it is popular or profitable, and regardless of the medium in which it appears."[7]

Jones agrees. In *Losing the News*, he wrote, "The profit squeeze has wreaked havoc on newsrooms and especially decimated the Washington-based press corps covering government on behalf of citizens back home."[8] Of greatest concern, Jones said, is the future of investigative journalism, which has the greatest value but costs the most to produce: "The problem is financial. A skilled investigative reporter can cost a news organization more than $250,000 a year in salary and expenses" and may produce just a handful of stories during that time.[9]

Meanwhile, the Occupational Employment Statistics Survey of May 2008, by the U.S. Bureau of Labor Statistics, showed 50,690 "reporter/correspondent" jobs in the country, with a mean annual income of $44,030. Correspondingly, there were 240,610 jobs for "public relations specialists," with a mean annual income of $58,960.[10]

With more and better-paying jobs available in PR than in journalism, fewer new college graduates are choosing to work in "iron core" news. It has been common historically for reporters to shift to PR after working as journalists, as I did. But it's a shocking development that a large percentage—actually a majority—of communications majors now opt to enter PR directly after college. These newly minted public relations practitioners begin their careers, in which they will be paid generously to pass off opinion and spin as "news," without first steeping themselves in the hard-and-fast rules of journalism and its ethics, which have provided a counterbalance to the worst instincts of many previous generations of public relations professionals.

"DOWN WITH NEWS, UP WITH SPIN"

Efforts to manipulate our opinions have grown increasingly pervasive over the last twenty years, in concert with the waning of traditional journalism. And with less access to credible information, we are more easily manipulated.

Göran Therborn, the renowned social theorist, author, and professor of sociology at Cambridge University, contends that there are three arguments most likely to sustain popular apathy toward any issue or problem: denying that the issue exists; insisting that it's a good thing rather than a bad thing; or conceding that it's a problem but claiming that it can't possibly be solved.[11]

All three have been used, with varying degrees of success, in the attempt to discredit the reality of global warming, despite the fact that an overwhelming majority of the world's scientists agree that the temperature of the earth is rising at a potentially disastrous rate as a direct result of human intervention in the planet's ecosystems.

In 1991, a consortium of fossil fuel energy associations established and funded a front group, which they named the Information Council for the Environment (with the clever-sounding acronym ICE). One of its major initiatives was the development of a half-million-dollar PR and advertising campaign to, in the words of ICE leadership, "reposition global warming as theory (not fact)."

Part of ICE's effort was to recruit sympathetic scientists, most of them from American universities, for a scientific advisory panel that would work to discredit the concept of global warming. Among the panel members was Patrick Michaels of the University of Virginia's Department of Environmental Services.

The plan was to use the media to publicize the views of the panelists—who were paid for their services—and a Washington-based PR agency arranged for print and broadcast interviews. Meanwhile, another firm conducted "public opinion polls," which targeted specific demographic groups (such as older males with limited education who were unlikely to seek additional information) and posed carefully crafted questions to illicit the desired responses. One of the resulting print ads carried the caption "Some say the earth is warming. Some also said the earth was flat." The accompanying graphic showed a sailing ship drifting toward a precipice—the outside edge of a flat earth. Beneath the drop sat a dragon, its mouth wide in anticipation of the falling ship.

The ICE campaign collapsed after someone leaked internal memos to the news media, among them a note from M. William Brier of the Edison Electric Institute, the trade association for U.S. shareholder-owned electric power companies, which included this sentence: "It will be interesting to see how the science approach sells."

The University of Virginia's Michaels rapidly parted ways with ICE at that point because of what he labeled as its "blatant dishonesty," although he continued to work with fossil fuel groups. In the midnineties, Michaels acknowledged that he had received $165,000 from fuel companies over the previous five years. He was also a paid expert witness for utility companies in lawsuits involving global warming issues and has also participated in anti-global-warming propaganda campaigns.[12]

In the new century, money from fossil fuel companies continues to perpetuate the American attachment to coal and petroleum, despite the undeniable benefits of shifting to renewable fuels and despite the growing public and political support for renewables like solar power. Brad Collins, the executive director of the American Solar Energy Society (ASES), wrote in early 2010, "At ASES, our job is to share our research and policy ideas with representatives doing the people's work. Many of our leaders, unfortunately, are overwhelmed by misinformation campaigns from the other side. The carbon lobby puts familiar faces into their offices far more often and with far more money than we can afford to do."[13]

OVERWHELMED OR UNDERINFORMED IN THE FUTURE

Rupert Murdoch's views on the future of American news are dramatically—and unsurprisingly—different from those of Arianna Huffington, the conservative-turned-liberal media powerhouse who cofounded the progressive Web site the Huffington Post. In a December 2009 speech that was reprinted on the site, Huffington predicted a "hybrid future where traditional media players embrace the ways of new media" and "new media companies adopt the best practices of old media."

She defended the "aggregation" of news (synopses or excerpts of stories with links to the original text) that Murdoch vehemently condemns. "This is a Golden Age for news consumers, who can search the Net, use search engines, access the best stories from around the world, and be able to comment, interact, and form communities. The value of having the world of information at your fingertips is beyond dispute," Huffington wrote.

In criticizing "traditional media companies" for putting profits ahead of modernizing their approach to news and "pleasing their readers," Huffington cited the following statistics:

- Newspaper circulation dropped by seven million in the last quarter century.
- "Unique" readership of online news increased by 34 percent in the last five years.
- Newspaper advertising declined by about 19 percent in 2009, while Internet advertising increased by 9 percent and mobile advertising grew by 18 percent.
- Internet users have access to more than one trillion Web pages.[14]

Huffington emphasized the generally accepted truth that traditional news organizations have yet to create a viable plan for charging for their online content to recoup some of the profits being lost to the Internet. She also roundly criticized news media for failing to fulfill their responsibilities to the public by "missing the two biggest stories of our time—the run-up to the war in Iraq and the financial meltdown." But she praised what she calls "new media journalists." "They're the true pit bulls of reporting," she wrote.

Huffington contends that the traditional definition of journalism is changing. News has "become something around which we gather, connect and converse," she wrote. "We all are part of the evolution of a story now—expanding it with comments and links to relevant information, adding facts and differing points of view." Newspapers, she said, are merely one piece of the journalistic pie: "We mustn't forget: The state of newspapers is not the same thing as the state of journalism. As much as I love newspapers—and fully expect them to survive—the future of journalism is not dependent on the future of newspapers."[15]

Huffington's decidedly optimistic take on new-media journalism implies that virtually everyone can function as an effective journalist and that objectivity and civic responsibility will rule Internet reporting. However, the sheer volume of information available online—together with the expanding efforts of the public relations industry to control both the content and the perspective of the "news" on behalf of its clients, as well as an understaffed, overwhelmed, and complicit news media—increasingly places the burden of responsibility on everyday Americans to distinguish real news from corporate spin.

Harvard's Jones cites the risks of relying on untrained journalists to be dependable sources of information, capable of replacing or supplementing the work of traditional newspeople. "The hollowed-out iron core of the future may well be mostly a compendium of the simplest, cheapest kind of bearing-witness whose job is to fill a quota of publishable copy rather than to cover a beat with depth," he wrote.[16]

It has come to this question: Can we afford to be reliant on even somewhat-accurate information provided by untrained observers at a time when professional efforts to manipulate information and reporting are increasingly successful?

There's also the unsettling effort to shout down legitimate traditional sources of news. Inflammatory, often outrageous rhetoric is used recklessly to inspire anger or even incite violence in an effort to gain financial or political power. Calculated dishonesty uses the news media as a whipping boy in order to instill mistrust of the "mainstream media" and turn audiences toward alternative, biased "news" sources with barely disguised agendas.

"To my mind, there *is* a genuine crisis," wrote Jones. "It is not one of press bias, though that is how most people seem to view it. Rather, it is a crisis of diminishing quantity and quality, of morale and sense of mission, of values and leadership. And it is taking place in a maelstrom of technological and economic change. The Internet and digital technology have sent the news business into a frenzy of rethinking, an upheaval of historic proportions whose outcome is much in doubt."[17]

Jones pointed out that each successive generation since World War II has relied less on newspapers, but today's young people seem to be turning away from objective information from any medium. "Young news consumers seem to greatly prefer news in a format that is anything but objective. Indeed, they seem to find objectivity not only dull, but less credible than someone who is apparently speaking his or her own mind. It does not seem to matter that such opinionated pronouncements may be claptrap and based on nothing but shallow knowledge."[18]

SPOTTING SPIN

The onslaughts will not stop, the distortions will not diminish, and the spin will not slow down. To the contrary, spin begets spin, as the successes of corporate PR functionaries increase the revenues of their employers, further funding their employers' efforts to create a more hospitable climate for their business interests. Americans are thus being faced with increasingly subtle but effective assaults on their beliefs and perceptions. Their best defense right now is to understand and to recognize the sophisticated tactics of the spinners trying to manipulate them. Most important is a singular mandate: Be skeptical.

The cliché that if it sounds too good to be true, it probably is, is generally true: The oil company that wants to reduce dependence on oil . . . the health insurance company that wants to make you well . . . the tobacco company that wants to discourage smoking . . . the finance company that wants to help you make money. Count on it: Any for-profit company that claims to have no self-interest has nothing *but*. Any for-profit company that claims to hold its customers' interests as paramount does so—if it actually does so—in order to keep those customers its own.

Knowing how to decode spin is as important as basic literacy and numeracy in today's media world.

As the previous chapters have demonstrated, and as I know from my own experience, many PR specialists attempt to reframe a public debate in order to shift the focus away from their client, introduce misleading information to dilute or redirect controversy, and use philanthropy as a way to overshadow negative publicity or questionable behavior on behalf of a corporation.

PR also spills over into advertising territory—paid time devoted to the promotion of an attitude rather than a product. Watch for ads that do not mention a specific item for sale but extol the virtues of a corporation and its contributions to society. Nary a negative word is spoken; there's simply an implicit message that this company is making your life better in some way. The idea is that if you hear the corporate name—the "brand"—enough, you'll equate it with the warm-and-fuzzy feelings of its messages and you'll buy whatever product is associated with it or, even more important, support the company when it's accused of lying to the public, or dumping toxic waste, or willfully marketing a product that causes more harm than good.

As I have pointed out, among the most prevalent and effective PR tactics is the "third-party technique," in which a supposedly disinterested individual or group throws support behind a cause, product, or candidate. For example, there's the Center for Consumer Freedom, which claims that its mission is to defend the rights of consumers to eat, drink, and smoke as they please. In reality, CCF is a front group for the tobacco, restaurant, and alcoholic beverage industries, which provide most of its funding.

Front groups often have Web sites, but they rarely provide a real physical address or a real phone number. If a Washington, D.C., address is provided, it is likely that of a lobbying organization or a PR firm. Front groups avoid mentioning their main funding sources, and they generally have misleading, feel-good names that stress patriotism, or individual freedom, or "American values."

To uncover the true nature of a front group, note the names of sponsoring groups. Check their Web sites and compare their physical addresses (if provided) and the names of staff members with those of lobbying and PR organizations—especially in Washington. Monitor SourceWatch (www.sourcewatch.org) for information on groups and individuals who have been identified as paid supporters of various corporations and causes.

WHAT IF?

Without basic knowledge of PR tactics and the ability to distinguish between fact and distortion, Americans—and that includes journalists, both professional and "citizen"—are at the mercy of spin doctors and public relations practitioners whose loyalty to their clients outweighs the public's right to the truth.

The Watergate scandal of the early 1970s, uncovered by two young reporters for the *Washington Post*, exposed the appalling activities, both unethical and illegal, of President Richard Nixon and his Committee to Re-Elect the President during the 1972 campaign. Not only does Watergate illustrate some of the most repugnant PR-type tactics—from using stolen stationery to issue fake announcements, to breaking into and bugging opponents' offices, to laundering money to cover the costs of the entire effort—but it also illustrates the critical role of a free and active press in our democracy. Nixon resigned in disgrace in 1974, and a cadre of his closest advisers and staff went to prison.

No one can know what would have happened if Bob Woodward

and Carl Bernstein of the *Post* had not been there to follow up on the break-in at the Watergate, but one thing's for sure: We need the Woodwards and Bernsteins of coming generations, regardless of the medium, to ensure that Americans have access to truth, and that a healthy balance between news and spin is in place.

Otherwise, our news will be coming—whether we know it or not—from companies with names like the Hawthorn Group, Edelman, Porter Novelli, and APCO Worldwide. If so, our way of life will be *truly* threatened.

Like Arianna Huffington, however, I'm an optimist.

I believe that one day the United States really will have one of the finest and most equitable health care systems in the world, and that insurance companies and banks and oil companies—in fact, all big corporations—will ultimately become more socially responsible.

People will demand it. It will take time and vigilance, but we can force even the biggest and most powerful corporations to be more honest and transparent in the way they do business and in the way they treat us, their customers, and in the way they treat our planet.

We will never be free of spin, but we can be wise to it, and we can push back against it. There is too much at stake not to try.

Acknowledgments

As I have thought about the many people I wanted to thank for helping me with this book, Stella Chambers and Bill Roesgen kept coming to mind. Mrs. Chambers, my senior year English teacher at Ketron High School in Kingsport, Tennessee, was the first person to suggest that I might be able to make a living as a writer. With her help, I landed my first job as a journalist, as Ketron's correspondent to the *Kingsport Times-News*, a newspaper that would play a big role four decades later in my decision to make a radical change in my life and career. I can't recall what I wrote about the goings on at Ketron that was deemed newsworthy, but somehow my dispatches attracted the attention of the paper's editor, Bill Roesgen, who hired me as a summer intern straight out of high school. I loved being a reporter so much that I decided to major in journalism when I got to the University of Tennessee. So thank you, Mrs. Chambers, and thank you, Bill Roesgen. I'm certain I would never have written this book if not for you.

There were many others who played a more direct role in the creation of *Deadly Spin*. I am especially indebted to a group of friends and former and current co-workers from my days in the newspaper business and, more recently, in the health insurance industry and at the Center for Media and Democracy. Thank you, Deborah Bowditch,

Barney DuBois, Avram Goldstein, Katie Hall, Anne Landman, and Dave MacHenry for helping me in the research and writing of the manuscript. Thanks also to my friend, former CIGNA colleague, and lawyer, Gabrielle Sellei. The many contributions you all made to the book were invaluable.

I am also indebted to Kirby Kim, my agent at William Morris Endeavor, and to the team at Bloomsbury Press who helped in the shaping, editing, and promotion of the book: Peter Ginna, George Gibson, Pete Beatty, Peter Miller, and Michelle Blankenship.

Long before I had the first thought of writing a book, many other people helped to make it inevitable that I would switch sides in the health care reform debate and become what many people have called a whistle-blower. Thank you especially Rev. Bill Golderer, Rev. Rodger Broadley, Rev. Michael Pergola, Joy Anderson, Rick Jacobs, Trudy Lieberman, Jonathan Cohn, Margie Maxwell, and Rob Scott for listening and asking the important questions I needed to answer for myself. Thank you Jamie Court, Michael Morrill, Len Nichols, Dr. Bob Crittenden, and Dr. Walter Tsou for helping me make important connections in the political and policy worlds. Thank you Richard Kirsch and your team at Health Care for America Now, especially Jacki Schechner, Doneg McDonough, Tara Straw, Ethan Rome, and, once again, Avram Goldstein, not only for the vital work you did to make sure that the bill Congress finally passed was worth passing but also for the support you gave me when I raised my hand to help in some way.

I had been a secret admirer of John Stauber and the Center for Media and Democracy, the organization John founded in 1993 to expose spin and propaganda, even while I was spinning for the insurance industry. Thank you, John, for being a flack's worst nightmare and for welcoming me to the CMD team as you were preparing to retire and hand the reins of the organization to the incomparable Lisa Graves. Thank you, Lisa, for the opportunity to work with you and learn from you and for the truly remarkable support you have given me. And thank you Nikolina Lazic, Page Metcalf, Sari Williams, and Mary Bottari at

CMD. I have never been a part of a team I have enjoyed more. I mean that sincerely.

Two other people I am especially grateful to are Sen. Jay Rockefeller of West Virginia, who afforded me the opportunity to testify before his Senate Commerce, Science, and Transportation Committee in what was to become my first of many public appearances as an industry critic and reform advocate, and to Bill Moyers, whose July 2009 interview with me on his *Bill Moyers Journal* on PBS made it possible for me to reach a national audience with my story.

Finally, thank you Stan Brock of Remote Area Medical and thank you, thank you, Nataline Sarkisyan. The world is a much better place because of you.

Resource Guide

Since I started speaking out about the abuses of the health insurance industry and explaining why Americans have put up with the most expensive and one of the most dysfunctional health care systems on the planet, countless people have asked me to intercede on their behalf with an insurance company that has refused to pay for care they need. Many others are among the 51 million Americans without coverage—or the 25 million who are underinsured. They've asked me if I can help them find decent coverage they can afford. Hundreds of people just want to know what they can do to make sure health care reform keeps going forward and how they can get involved in the fight for a more rational and equitable system. More than a few have asked me to explain how the Affordable Care Act, which President Obama signed into law on March 23, 2010, will affect them and their families.

I wish I could help them all and answer everyone's questions individually. Since that's not possible, I decided to compile a list of resources for this paperback edition of *Deadly Spin*. As you'll see, it runs the gamut from useful government Web sites to unions and advocacy groups. At the very top of the list is a site that gets better just about every day: www.healthcare.gov. Created and constantly updated by the U.S. Department of Health and Human Services (HHS), the site would not be possible if the health care reform law had not been enacted.

Few people realize it, but the law requires health insurers and health care providers to provide much more information than they've ever disclosed in the past. HHS is not only compiling all this new information, but it's also making it available in ways that enable consumers to make comparisons among insurers and providers with just a few clicks of a mouse. I encourage you to become a regular visitor to the site.

I also encourage you to get involved and stay involved in the ongoing battle for a health care system that meets the needs of all Americans. The Affordable Care Act was a start, but it is just that: a start. I call it the end of the beginning of reform. You will find many organizations, at both the state and national levels that will welcome your participation.

One last bit of advice: If your insurance company denies you coverage for care your doctor says you need, don't take that as a final decision. You have rights—including some new ones under the Affordable Care Act—that you should know about and exercise. Go to www .healthcare.gov and explore some of the other resources listed below to learn more about them. At the very least, start the appeals process. Insurers know that most people give up because they don't know their rights or are intimidated at the very thought of trying to get a denial reversed. If you're not well enough to do it yourself, ask a friend or family member to help or contact one or more of the organizations in this resource guide and ask if they can advocate on your behalf.

Above all, be a squeaky wheel if you're getting the runaround from your insurer. Don't just call the member services number on your ID card. Get the main number for your insurance company and call it, demanding to speak to the CEO. You won't get him or her on the line, but you will get somebody's attention. Tell them you plan to take your case to the media and your elected state and federal representatives. If you've done that already, tell them so. If you haven't, do it. Contact a consumer reporter at a local TV station and a health care reporter at your newspaper. They might take a pass on your story, but nothing ventured, nothing gained. Give it a shot. And take your case to your state legislators and members of Congress, They work for you.

Make sure they all know your name. Be a pest if necessary. Remember, the only wheels that get any grease are the squeaky ones.

If you read about or see an advertisement sponsored by an organization you've never heard of before and wonder who is behind it, go to www.SourceWatch.org, a "collaborative resource for citizens and journalists looking for documented information about the corporations, industries, and people trying to sway public opinion." Two other excellent sites created to help people sort truth from fiction are www .FactCheck.org and www.PolitiFact.org. FactCheck.org, a project of the Annenberg Public Policy Center of the University of Pennsylvania, "monitors the factual accuracy of what is said by major U.S. political players in the form of TV ads, debates, speeches, interviews and news releases." PolitiFact.com is a project of the *St. Petersburg Times* "to help you find the truth in politics." Reporters and researchers at the newspaper "examine statements by members of Congress, the president, cabinet secretaries, lobbyists, people who testify before Congress and anyone else who speaks up in Washington." PolitiFact.com rates the accuracy of the statements it examines on its Truth-O-Meter. The most ridiculous falsehoods get the lowest rating, Pants on Fire.

GOVERNMENT AND QUASI-GOVERNMENT SOURCES

HealthCare.gov (www.healthcare.gov) is an official government Web site that provides information on finding insurance options, comparing care quality, and understanding the new health care reform law. It also has a section of frequently asked questions.

HealthFinder.gov (www.healthfinder.gov) is another excellent government site that provides an encyclopedia of more than sixteen hundred health topics as well as interactive tools to check your health and get personal advice.

Medicare.gov (www.medicare.gov) is the official government site for Medicare beneficiaries. It provides information on Medicare billing, enrollment, benefits, discount drug cards, and long-term care. The site also includes a glossary of terms and a variety of search tools to help enrollees compare health plan options, locate participating physicians, and compare nursing homes.

Medline Plus (www.nlm.nih.gov/medlineplus) makes available information from the National Library of Medicine (NLM), the National Institutes of Health (NIH), and other government agencies and health-related organizations. It also provides access to medical journal articles and has extensive information about drugs, an illustrated medical encyclopedia, interactive patient tutorials, and current health news.

Federal Citizen Information Center (FCIC) (www.pueblo.gsa .gov; 888-878-3256) answers questions about federal agencies, programs, and services, and provides access to hundreds of consumer publications.

National Association of Insurance Commissioners (www.naic .org; 816-783-8500) assists state insurance regulators "in serving the public interest." The site also contains useful information for consumers and a list of state insurance commissioners (www.naic.org/documents/members_membershiplist.pdf).

Rural Assistance Center (www.raconline.org; 800-270-1898), a project of the U.S. Department of Health and Human Services, helps rural communities and other rural stakeholders gain access to a broad range of available programs, funding, and research that can enable them to provide health and human services to rural residents.

CONSUMER-INTEREST GROUPS

AARP (www.aarp.org; 888-687-2277) offers information on housing, insurance, eligibility for public benefits, financial security, transportation, and consumer protection issues on behalf of midlife and older consumers.

American Cancer Society (www.cancer.org; 800-227-2345) is a nationwide, community-based voluntary health organization dedicated to eliminating cancer as a major health problem.

American Heart Association (www.heart.org; 800-242-8721) is a national voluntary health agency whose mission is to reduce disability and death from cardiovascular diseases and stroke.

American Diabetes Association (www.diabetes.org; 800-342-2383) is a national organization whose mission is to prevent and cure diabetes and to improve the lives of people affected by the disease.

Autism Speaks (www.autismspeaks.org; 888-288-4962) is the nation's largest autism science and advocacy organization, dedicated to funding research into the causes, prevention, treatments, and cure for autism.

Better Business Bureau (BBB) (www.bbb.org/us/consumers; 703-276-0100) offers a variety of consumer services, including educational materials, information on charities and other organizations seeking public donations, and mediation and arbitration services.

Coalition Against Insurance Fraud (www.insurancefraud.org; 202-393-7330) is an organization of consumers, government agencies, and insurers "dedicated to combating all forms of insurance fraud."

Consumers Union (CU) (www.consumersunion.org; 914-378-2000) is an independent, nonprofit organization "whose mission is to work for a fair, just, and safe marketplace for all consumers and to empower consumers to protect themselves." CU created ConsumerReports Health.org and the Consumer Reports Health Ratings Center, which provides comparisons of health services, drugs, devices, and consumer experiences, "to educate and empower consumers to make more informed health-care decisions and to help change the market."

Consumer Watchdog (www.consumerwatchdog.org; 310-392-0522) is a nonprofit organization "dedicated to providing an effective voice for taxpayers and consumers . . . [and] taking on politicians of both parties and the special interests that fund them."

Families USA (www.familiesusa.org; 202-628-3030) is a national nonprofit, nonpartisan advocacy organization "dedicated to the achievement of high-quality, affordable health care for all Americans." Its site also provides an extensive list of research organizations and state-based advocacy groups (www.familiesusa.org/resources/related -links/).

Health Insurance Info (www.healthinsurance.net; 202-687-0880), a project of the Georgetown University Health Policy Institute, provides online consumer guides for each state and the District of Columbia. It also provides summaries of laws that have been enacted "to protect people when they are trying to get and keep health insurance."

Medicare Rights Center (www.medicarerights.org; 800-333-4114) is a national, nonprofit consumer service organization that works to ensure access to affordable health care for older adults and people with disabilities through counseling and advocacy, educational programs, and public policy initiatives.

National Alliance on Mental Illness (www.nami.org; 800-950-6264) is a grassroots mental health advocacy organization.

National Consumers League (nclnet.org; 202-835-3323), founded in 1899, bills itself as "America's pioneer consumer advocacy organization." It focuses on consumer health and safety protection as well as fairness in the marketplace and workplace.

National Council on Aging (www.ncoa.org; 800-677-1116) advocates on behalf of older adults and community organizations that serve them.

National Multiple Sclerosis Society (www.nationalmssociety.org; 800-344-4867) is a nationwide organization with chapters in all fifty states that provides education programs and furthers MS advocacy and research.

National Senior Citizens Law Center (www.nsclc.org; 202-289-6976) advocates for people with limited resources and income and provides them with access to the judicial system.

Public Citizen (www.citizen.org; 202-588-1000) represents consumer interests in Congress, the courts, government agencies, and the media. Its divisions include Auto Safety, Congress Watch, Critical Mass (Energy & Environment Program), Global Trade Watch, the Health Research Group, and the Litigation Group.

NATIONAL ADVOCACY AND CONSUMER GROUPS AND UNIONS

Alliance for a Just Society (www.allianceforajustsociety.org; 206-568-5400) is a national organization whose affiliates are member-based groups representing low-income people, immigrants, and people of color. The Alliance "is committed to advancing racial and economic justice and, with its partners in the 24-state Health Rights Organizing Project, is a leader in the fight to address racial and ethnic disparities through health reform."

Grass Roots Organizing (GRO) (www.gromo.org; 877-581-9595) is a membership-driven social justice organization. GRO works to "hold corporate America accountable and advance health care for all, housing rights, food security and other social-economic justice reforms."

Health Care for America Now (HCAN) (www.healthcareforamerica now.org; 202-454-6200) is "a national grassroots campaign of more than 1,000 organizations in 46 states representing 30 million people dedicated to winning quality, affordable health care." A leading advocate of federal health care reform, it is now focused on implementing and improving comprehensive health care reform by helping people become citizen lobbyists.

Health Care Now! (www.healthcare-now.org; 800-453-1305) is a grassroots organization with organizers and activists in more than three hundred cities in all fifty states that addresses the health insurance crisis in the U.S. by educating and advocating for the passage of single-payer health care legislation.

Main Street Alliance (www.mainstreetalliance.org; 603-831-1835) is a national network of small business coalitions. "MSA creates opportunities for small business owners to speak for themselves on issues that impact their businesses, their employees, and local economies."

National Education Association (www.nea.org; 202-833-4000) represents educators throughout the country as well as at U.S. facilities around the world that. Among other things, the organization "advocates for quality, comprehensive, and affordable health care" to ensure that "educators and their students come to school ready to work and ready to learn."

Physicians for a National Health Program (www.pnhp.org; 312-782-6006) is a nonprofit research and education organization of eighteen thousand physicians, medical students, and health professionals who support single-payer national health insurance.

Service Employees International Union (SEIU) (www.seiu.org; 800-424-8592) is a 2.2 million-member organization "dedicated to improving the lives of workers and their families and creating a more just and humane society . . . SEIU members built a national movement over more than a decade to support the passage of a health care law that would ensure that everyone in America had access to quality, affordable health care."

USAction (www.usaction.org; 202-263-4520) is a federation of twenty-four state affiliates and partners "that organize for a more just America." (USAction also cofounded Health Care for America Now and serves as cochair of its steering committee).

Young Invincibles (www.younginvincibles.org; 202-339-9338) is a national organization founded to educate, inform, and represent the interests of eighteen- to thirty-four-year-olds in health care reform.

STATE-BASED ADVOCACY AND CONSUMER GROUPS

Alabama
Health Care for Everyone Alabama (www.healthcareforeveryone -alabama.org; 205-930-3774)

Alaska
Alaska Center for Public Policy (www.acpp.info; 907-276-2277)

Arizona
Living United for Change in Arizona (www.luchaaz.org; 602-388-9745)

Arkansas
Arkansas Community Organizations (www.arkansascomm.org; 501-376-7151)

California
California OneCare (www.californiaonecare.org; 888-442-4255)

California Partnership (www.california-partnership.org; 213-385-8010)

Health Access California (www.health-access.org; 916-497-0923)

Colorado
Colorado Consumer Health Initiative (www.cohealthinitiative .org; 303-839-1261)

Colorado Progressive Action (www.coprogressiveaction.org; 303-863-8390)

Connecticut
Connecticut Citizen Action Group (www.ccag.net; 860-233-2181)

United Action Connecticut (www.uact4justice.org; 860-882-3849)

Delaware
Delaware Health Care Commission (www.dhss.delaware.gov/dhss/ dhcc; 302-739-2730)

Florida
Florida Consumer Action Network (www.fcan.org; 813-877-6712)

Georgia
Georgians for a Healthy Future (www.healthyfuturega.org; 404-567-5016)

Hawaii
Hawaii Coalition for Health (www.h-c4h.org; 808-622-2655)

Illinois
Citizen Action/Illinois (www.citizenaction-il.org; 312-427-2114)

Iowa
Iowa Citizen Action Network (www.Iowacan.org; 515-277-5077)

Maine
Maine People's Alliance (www.mainepeoplesalliance.org; 207-797-0967)

Maryland
Progressive Maryland (www.progressivemaryland.org; 301-495-7004)

Massachusetts
Massachusetts Public Interest Research Group (www.masspirg .org; 617-292-4800)

Massachusetts Health Care for All (www.hcfama.org; 617-350-7279)

Michigan
Michigan Citizen Action (www.michcitizenaction.org; 269-349-9170)

Progress Michigan (www.progressmichigan.org; 517-999-3646)

Minnesota
TakeAction Minnesota (www.takeactionminnesota.org; 651-641-6199)

Missouri
Cover Missouri (www.covermissouri.org; 314-345-5574)

Montana
Montana Organizing Project (www.montanaorganizingproject.org; 406-529-8497)

Nebraska
Nebraska Appleseed Center for Law in the Public Interest (http://neappleseed.org; 800-845-3746)

Nevada
Progressive Leadership Alliance of Nevada (www.planevada.org; 702-791-1965)

New Hampshire
New Hampshire Citizens Alliance (www.nhcitizensalliance.org; 603-225-2097)

New Jersey
New Jersey Citizen Action (www.njcitizenaction.org; 973-643-8800)

New Mexico
Health Action New Mexico (www.healthactionnm.org; 877-867-1095)

New York
Citizen Action of New York (www.citizenactionny.org; 518-465-4600)

Health Care for All New York (www.hcfany.org; 212-614-5401)

North Carolina
Action NC (www.actionnc.org; 704-625-4050)

North Carolina Social Justice Project (www.ncsjp.org; 919-295-2870)

North Dakota
NDPeople.org (www.ndpeople.org; 701-527-0060)

Ohio
ProgressOhio (www.progressohio.org; 614-441-9144)

Oregon
Oregon State Public Interest Research Group (OSPIRG) (www.ospirg.org; 503-231-4181)

Pennsylvania
Keystone Progress (www.keystoneprogress.org; 610-990-6300)

Penn ACTION (www.pennaction.org; 215-880-6142)

The Pennsylvania Health Access Network (http://pahealthaccess .org; 215-557-0822)

Rhode Island
Ocean State Action (www.oceanstateaction.org; 401-463-5368)

Tennessee
Tennessee Citizen Action (www.tnca.org; 615-736-6040)

Tennessee Health Care Campaign (www.tenncare.org; 877-431-7083)

Tennessee Justice Center (www.tnjustice.org; 877-608-1009)

Texas
Center for Public Policy Priorities (www.cppp.org; 512-320-0222)

Utah
Utah Health Policy Project (www.healthpolicyproject.org; 801-433-2299)

Vermont
Vermont Public Interest Research Group (www.vpirg.org; 802-223-5221)

Vermont Workers' Center (www.workerscenter.org; 802-861-4892)

Virginia
Virginia Organizing (www.virginia-organizing.org; 434-984-4655)

Washington
Washington Community Action Network (www.washingtoncan .org; 206-389-0050)

West Virginia
West Virginia Citizen Action Group (www.wvcag.org; 304-346-5891)

Wisconsin
Citizen Action of Wisconsin (http://citizenactionwi.org; 414-476-4501)

Wyoming
Equality State Policy Center (www.equalitystate.org; 307-472-5939)

Notes

INTRODUCTION

1. *Taking the Risk out of Democracy: Propaganda in the U.S. and Australia*, Alex Carey, University of New South Wales Press, 1995.
2. Karen Ignagni, president of America's Health Insurance Plans (AHIP), White House, March 5, 2009.
3. "Health Insurance and Mortality in U.S. Adults," Andrew P. Wilper et al., *American Journal of Public Health*, December 2009, 99: 2289–95.
4. *The Hidden Persuaders*, Vance Packard, David McKay Company, 1957, 32.
5. *The Invisible Persuaders*, David Michie, Bantam Press, 1998.

CHAPTER III: PERCEPTION IS REALITY

1. *Cutlip & Center's Effective Public Relations*, Glen M. Broom, Prentiss Hall, 2009, 3.
2. Public Relations Society of America, http://www.prsa.org/AboutPRSA/PublicRelationsDefined.
3. *Toxic Sludge Is Good for You*, John Stauber and Sheldon Rampton, Common Courage Press, 1995, 17.
4. *The Unseen Power: Public Relations—A History*, Scott M. Cutlip, Lawrence Erlbaum Associates, 1994, 52–53, 97.
5. *The Father of Spin*, Larry Tye, Henry Holt and Company, 1998, ix.
6. Ibid., 23–31.
7. *Toxic Sludge*, Stauber and Rampton, 292–94.
8. Public Relations Society of America, http://www.prsa.org/AboutPRSA.

9. Franco did not admit to or deny the charges but did enter into an agreement with the SEC not to violate the agency's regulations in the future.

10. "Wal-Mart Stores Inc.: Publicist Enlists Bloggers to Combat Negative News," *Wall Street Journal*, March 7, 2006.

11. "Wal-Mart vs. the Blogosphere," Pallavi Gogoi, BusinessWeek.com, Oct. 18, 2006, accessed at http://www.msnbc.msn.com/id/15319926.

12. "Book of Tens: Agencies of the Decade," *Advertising Age*, Dec. 14, 2009, accessed at http://www.edelman.com/news/2010/Ad_Age_AgencyAList.pdf.

13. *Toxic Sludge*, Stauber and Rampton, 6–8.

14. *Propaganda*, Edward Bernays, Ig Publishing, 2005, 37.

15. *The Biography of an Idea: Memoirs of Public Relations Counsel Edward L. Bernays*, Simon and Schuster, 1965, 652.

16. *Mein Kampf*, Adolf Hitler, vol. 2, *A Reckoning*, chap. 6, "War Propaganda," accessed at http://www.hitler.org/writings/Mein_Kampf/mkv1ch06.html.

17. *The Later Years: Public Relations Insights 1956–1986*, Edward L. Bernays, Howard Pen Hudson Associates, 1986, 115.

18. *Later Years*, Bernays, 139.

19. *Effective Public Relations*, Broom, 25.

CHAPTER IV: REMOTE AREA MEDICAL IN WISE COUNTY, VIRGINIA

1. *How to Lie with Statistics*, Darrell Huff, W. W. Norton & Company, 1952, 100–121.

2. "Changes in Health Insurance Coverage, 2007–2008: Early Impact of the Recession," Kaiser Commission on Medicaid and the Uninsured, October 2009.

3. "Average Family Health Insurance Policy: $13,375, Up 5%," *USA Today*, Sept. 16, 2009.

4. "Employers, Workers, and the Future of Employment-Based Health Benefits," Employee Benefits Research Institute, February 2010.

5. "More Small Firms Drop Health Care," *Wall Street Journal*, May 26, 2009.

6. "Behind Aetna's Turnaround: Small Steps to Pare Cost of Care," *Wall Street Journal*, Aug. 13, 2004.

CHAPTER V: HEALTH CARE HISTORY, REFORM, AND FAILURE

1. http://www.youtube.com/watch?v=fRdLpem-AAs.

2. *PBS Newshour*, March 30, 2007.

3. *The Social Transformation of American Medicine*, Paul Starr, Basic Books, 1982, 237.

4. Ibid., 243.

5. *One Nation Uninsured: Why the U.S. Has No National Health Insurance*, Jill Quadagno, Oxford University Press, 2005, 17.

6. Ibid., 19.

7. *Social Transformation*, Starr, 253.

8. The Blue Shield plans, which initially only provided coverage for medical care provided by physicians, developed separately from Blue Cross plans, which in their early years only covered hospital care. The first Blue Shield plan was organized in California in 1939.

9. *Social Transformation*, Starr, 261–66.

10. *One Nation Uninsured*, Quadagno, 23.

11. *Critical: What We Can Do About the Health-Care Crisis*, Senator Tom Daschle, Thomas Dunne Books, 2008, 49.

12. *Social Transformation*, Starr, 277.

13. *Critical*, Daschle, 51.

14. Ibid., 52.

15. *Social Transformation*, Starr, 285.

16. *Critical*, Daschle, 53.

17. Ibid.

18. Ibid., 59.

19. Ibid., 63.

20. *Social Transformation*, Starr, 381.

21. *One Nation Uninsured*, Quadagno, 116.

CHAPTER VI: CONSUMER-DRIVEN CARE

1. "How Many Are Underinsured? Trends Among U.S. Adults, 2003 and 2007," Cathy Schoen et al., *Health Affairs*, June 2008. Respondents to the Commonwealth Fund survey were identified as underinsured if they spent 10 percent or more of their income (or 5 percent if they were low-income) on out-of-pocket medical expenses, or if they had deductibles that equaled 5 percent or more of their income.

2. "Health Care Access Problems Surge Among Insured Americans," Doug Trapp *American Medical News*, July 21, 2008.

3. "CIGNA Ex-CEO Hanway's Retirement Payments Near $111 Million," *Wall Street Journal*, March 19, 2010.

4. *The Great Risk Shift*, Jacob S. Hacker, Oxford University Press, 2006, 37.

5. "CIGNA Choice Fund (SM) Study Provides New Insights on Consumer Decision-Making in Consumer-Driven Health Plans," http://newsroom.cigna .com/article_display.cfm?article_id=669.

6. "Healthier, Wealthier and Wiser? An Overview of Consumer-Driven Health Care," Roberta W. Goodman, UnitedHealth Group, 2005.
7. PricewaterhouseCoopers news release, July 18, 2005.
8. "Workers May Be in for Health Plan Sticker Shock," *USA Today*, Oct. 21, 2005.

CHAPTER VII: IT'S ALL ABOUT THE MONEY

1. "What Happened to Health Care Reform?" Paul Starr, *American Prospect*, Winter 1995, 20–31.
2. "The Demise of the Clinton Plan," Theda Skocpol, *Health Affairs*, Spring 1995, 66–85.
3. "National Health Expenditure Data," Center for Medicare and Medicaid Services, accessed at http://www.cms.gov/NationalHealthExpendData/downloads/tables.pdf.
4. "Lost Cause," Peter H. Stone, *National Journal*, September 1994.
5. "Killing Health Care Reform," Thomas Scarlett, *Politics*, October/November 1994, 34.
6. "Shaping Public Opinion: If You Don't Do It, Somebody Else Will," Blair Childs, seminar, Chicago, Dec. 9, 1994.
7. *Toxic Sludge Is Good for You*, John Stauber and Sheldon Rampton, Common Courage Press, 1995, 96.
8. *My Life*, William Jefferson Clinton, Alfred A. Knopf, 2004, 62.
9. "Demise," Skocpol, 66–85.
10. Ibid.
11. "What the For-Profit Trend in Health Care Really Means," Paul Wynn, *Managed Care*, June 1996, accessed at http://www.managedcaremag.com/archives/9606/MC9606.profit.shtml.
12. "Nonprofit Health Insurers: The Financial Story Wall Street Doesn't Tell," Susan R. Barrish, Alliance for Advancing Nonprofit HealthCare," accessed at http://www.healthleadersmedia.com/pdf/white_papers/wp_alliance_011904.pdf.
13. "Kathleen Sebelius," WhoRunsGov.com, http://www.whorunsgov.com/profiles/kathleen_sebelius.
14. "CareFirst Sale Rejected by Md. Insurance Commissioner," Jo Becker, *Washington Post*, March 6, 2003, accessed at http://www.carefirstwatch.com/news/news.cfm?ID=41.
15. "CEO Total Compensation for Selected Blue Cross-Blue Shields, U.S. Medicare Program, 2007," Health Care for America Now.
16. Testimony of David Balto, senior fellow, Center for American Progress Action Fund, before the U.S. House of Representatives, Judiciary Committee, Subcommittee on Courts and Competition Policy, on H.R. 3596, Health Insurance Industry Antitrust Enforcement Act of 2009, accessed at http://judiciary.house.gov/hearings/pdf/Balto091008.pdf.

17. "AMA Study Shows Competition Disappearing in the Health Insurance Industry," American Medical Association, Feb. 23, 2010, accessed at http://www.ama-assn.org/ama/pub/news/news/health-insurance-competition.shtml.

18. "Premiums Soaring in Consolidated Health Insurance Market: Lack of Competition Hurts Rural States, Small Businesses," Health Care for America Now, May 2009, accessed at http://hcfan.3cdn.net/1b741c44183247e6ac_2om6i6nzc.pdf.

19. "A Handshake That Made Healthcare History," Globe Spotlight Team, *Boston Globe*, December 28, 2008, accessed at http://www.boston.com/news/health/articles/2008/12/28/a_handshake_that_made_healthcare_history.

20. "Premiums Soaring," Health Care for America Now.

21. "UnitedHealth CEO McGuire Gives Back $620 Million," Peter Lattman, *Wall Street Journal*, Dec. 7, 2007, accessed at http://blogs.wsj.com/law/2007/12/07/unitedhealth-ceo-mcguires-gives-back-620-million.

22. Securities and Exchange Commission filings.

23. "The Explosion of Executive Pay and the Erosion of American Prosperity," William Lazonick, University of Massachusetts Lowell and Université Montesquieu-Bordeaux IV, Feb. 24, 2010.

24. "Medical Benefit Ratios of Private Insurers, Public Medicare Plan, 1993 to 2007," Health Care for America Now, October 2010, accessed at http://hcfan.3cdn.net/15b2e716998ad2bddo_ktm6bz8uo.pdf.

25. "Health Insurers Falsely Claim Rising Costs Justify Soaring Premiums," Health Care for America Now, March 2010, accessed at http://hcfan.3cdn.net/578b1f7456962bfa7a_r6m6bhcjn.pdf.

26. Ibid.

27. Securities and Exchange Commission filings.

28. "Report to the Congress: Medicare Payment Policy," Medicare Payment Advisory Commission, March 2009, accessed at http://www.medpac.gov/documents/Mar09_EntireReport.pdf.

29. "A Scrappy Insurer Wrestles with Reform," Reed Abelson, *New York Times*, May 16, 2010.

CHAPTER IX: ERISA STYMIES THE SARKISYANS, AND US

1. "ERISA: Barrier to Health Care Consumers' Rights," National Association of Insurance Commissioners, 2000.

2. *Making a Killing: HMOs and the Threat to Your Health*, Jamie Court and Francis Smith, Common Courage Press, 1999, 122.

3. "Employee Health Plan Protections Under ERISA," Karl Polzer, *Health Affairs*, September/October 1997, 93–102.

4. For more information about Nataline's Legacy Fashion Show, contact Hilda Sarkisyan at hildasarkisyan@realtor.com.

CHAPTER X: A VICTORY, OF SORTS

1. "Obamarama," *Chicago Reader*, March 17, 2000, accessed at http://www1.chi cagoreader.com/obama/000317.

2. "Did Obama Campaign on Public Option?" Mark Murray and Domenico Montanaro, MSNBC, Dec. 23, 2009, accessed at http://firstread.msnbc.msn .com/archive/2009/12/23/2159620.aspx. Also see "Did Obama Campaign on the Public Option? Yes but Not Entirely," Sam Stein, Huffington Post, Dec. 22, 2009, http://www.huffingtonpost.com/2009/12/22/did-obama-campaign -on-the_n_401204.html.

3. "Obama Proposes $634 Billion Fund for Health Care," Ceci Connolly, *Washington Post*, Feb. 26, 2009, accessed at http://www.washingtonpost.com/wp-dyn/con tent/article/2009/02/25/AR2009022502587.html.

4. "Karen Ignagni," WhoRunsGov.com, http://www.whorunsgov.com/Profiles/ Karen_Ignagni.

5. "Fat Paydays for Key Players on Both Sides of Health Care Debate," Justin El-liott, Talking Points Memo, March 18, 2010, http://tpmmuckraker.talkingpoints memo.com/2010/03/health_care_lobby_players_fat_pay_days.php.

6. "Unlikely Lobbyist Will Lead H.M.O.'s into Battle," Robert Pear, *New York Times*, July 12, 1999, accessed at http://www.nytimes.com/1999/07/12/us/un likely-lobbyist-will-lead-hmo-s-into-battle.html?sec=health&spon=&page wanted=all.

7. "Insurance and HMO Industries Spend Nearly $700,000 per Day to Kill Health Care Reform Measures," Public Campaign Action Fund, Sept. 15, 2009, accessed at http://www.campaignmoney.org/HMO_insurance_spend_to_kill_ reform.

8. "The Case for Public Plan Choice in National Health Reform: Key to Cost Control and Quality Coverage," Jacob S. Hacker, Ph.D., Institute for America's Future, Dec. 16, 2008, accessed at http://institute.ourfuture.org/files/Jacob_ Hacker_Public_Plan_Choice.pdf?#.

9. "Poll: Most Back Public Health Care Option," CBS News, June 20, 2009, ac-cessed at http://www.cbsnews.com/stories/2009/06/19/opinion/polls/main5098517 .shtml.

10. "National Health Expenditures Historicals for 1960–2007," table 13, Centers for Medicare and Medicaid Services, U.S. Department of Health and Human Services, accessed at http://www.cms.hhs.gov/NationalHealthExpendData/ downloads/tables.pdf.

11. "Insurer-Owned Consulting Firm Often Cited in Health Debate," David Hil-zenrath, *Washington Post*, July 23, 2009, Accessed at http://www.washington post.com/wp-dyn/content/article/2009/07/22/AR2009072203696.html.

12. "The Health Insurers Have Already Won," Chad Terhune and Keith Epstein, *BusinessWeek*, Aug. 6, 2009, accessed at http://www.businessweek.com/maga zine/content/09_33/b4143034820260.htm.

13. "Health Care: It's Time for a Major Overhaul," Alexander Zaitchik, AlterNet, Dec. 1, 2008, http://www.alternet.org/story/109230.

14. "Top Insurance Lobbyist: Dem 'Vilification' Could Kill Reform," Alan Fram, Associated Press, Aug. 10, 2009, accessed at http://www.huffingtonpost.com/2009/08/10/karen-ignagni-ahip-presid_n_255615.html.

15. "Reality Check: AHIP's 'Study' Hard to Take Seriously," White House Blog, Oct. 12, 2009, http://www.whitehouse.gov/blog/Reality-Check-AHIPs-Study-Hard-to-Take-Seriously.

16. "PricewaterhouseCoopers Backs Away from AHIP," Ezra Klein, *Washington Post*, Oct. 13, 2009, accessed at http://voices.washingtonpost.com/ezra-klein/2009/10/pricewaterhousecoopers_backs_a.html.

17. "Prognosis Improves for Public Insurance," Shailagh Murray and Lori Montgomery, *Washington Post*, Oct. 24, 2009, accessed at http://www.washingtonpost.com/wp-dyn/content/article/2009/10/23/AR2009102304081.html?sid=ST2009102400183.

18. "Anthem Blue Cross Dramatically Raising Rates for Californians with Individual Health Policies," Duke Helfand, *Los Angeles Times*, Feb. 4, 2010, accessed at http://articles.latimes.com/2010/feb/04/business/la-fi-insure-anthem5-2010feb05.

CHAPTER XI: THE PLAYBOOK

1. "Tobacco Additives: Cigarette Engineering & Nicotine Addiction," Clive Bates, Martin Jarvis, and Gregory Connolly, Action on Smoking and Health, July 14, 1999.

2. Document 2075733345/3346, Philip Morris Collection (hereafter "PM"), 2000, Legacy Tobacco Documents Library (hereafter "LTDL"), http://legacy.library.ucsf.edu.

3. "Enzi: Peace Treaty with Philip Morris No Way to Win War on Tobacco," TradingMarkets.com, May 21, 2009, http://www.tradingmarkets.com/.site/news/Stock%20News/2340845.

4. Document 2501358202/8212, PM, 1994, LTDL, http://legacy.library.ucsf.edu.

5. Document 505467389/7392, R. J. Reynolds Collection (hereafter "RJR"), 1986, LTDL, http://legacy.library.ucsf.edu.

6. Document 2047871256/1259, LTDL, http://legacy.library.ucsf.edu.

7. Document 507746564/6567, RJR, 1991, LTDL, http://legacy.library.ucsf.edu.

8. Document 2023959567/9579, LTDL, http://legacy.library.ucsf.edu.

9. "Pro-Tobacco Writer Admits He Should Have Declared an Interest," Zosia Kmietowicz and Annabel Ferriman, *British Medical Journal*, February 2002; also Document 208578334/3335, LTDL, 2002, http://legacy.library.ucsf.edu/tid/rce20c00.

10. "A Snort of Derision," Roger Scruton, *Times* (United Kingdom), October 19, 1998; also Document 2064822424-2426, LTDL, http://legacy.library.ucsf.edu.

11. Document 2504092395/2405, LTDL, http://legacy.library.ucsf.edu.
12. Document 2025492898/2905, PM, 1994, LTDL, http://legacy.library.ucsf.edu.
13. Document 2024233677/3682, LTDL, http://legacy.library.ucsf.edu.
14. "How BP Secretly Buys PR," Rick Outzen, Daily Beast, May 19, 2010, http:www.thedailybeast.com/blogs-and-stories/2010-05-19/how-bp-secretly-buys-pr/.
15. "Slick Operator: How British Oil Giant BP Used All the Political Muscle Money Can Buy to Fend Off Regulators and Influence Investigations into Corporate Neglect," Michael Isikoff and Michael Hirsh, *Newsweek*, May 7, 2010.
16. "BP: Coloring Public Opinion," Gregory Solman, *Adweek*, Jan. 14, 2008.
17. "Oil Industry Front Group Runs Climate Change Disinfo Ads," David Gutierrez, NaturalNews.com, Sept. 7, 2009, www.naturalnews.com/026985_oil_industry_climate_change_natural_health.html.
18. "The 700 Club," Jake Whitney, Guernica, April 26, 2010, www.guernicamag.com/interviews/1687/700_club/.
19. "Lobbyists Lining Up Against Nutter's Soda Tax," Jeff Shields, *Philadelphia Inquirer*, March 11, 2010.
20. "Soda Tax Gone; Nutter Eyes Jobs," Catherine Lucey, *Philadelphia Daily News*, May 21, 2010.
21. "D.C. Soda Tax Proposal Draws Opposition from Beverage Industry," Tim Craig, *Washington Post*, May 14, 2010.
22. "Rent-A-Front: New Group Wages Stealth Battle Against Wall Street Reform," Justin Elliott, Talking Points Memo, April 21, 2010, www.tpmmuckraker.talkingpointsmemo.com/2010/04/rent-a-front_stop_too_big_to_fail_fights_reform.php.
23. "Goldman Sachs Publicly Supports Financial Reform, but Fights It with Lobbyists," Adele Hampton, Huffington Post, May 17, 2010, www.huffingtonpost.com/2010/05/17/goldman-sachs-publicly-su_n_578434.html.

CHAPTER XII: SPINNING OUT OF CONTROL

1. *Losing the News*, Alex S. Jones, Oxford University Press, 2009, 221.
2. "Murdoch Sees Newspaper Future on iPads," Sylvia Smith, NPC Wire, April 7, 2010, accessed at http://www.press.org/wire/article.cfm?id=2059.
3. "Rocky Mountain News to Close, Publish Final Edition Friday," Lynn DeBruin, *Rocky Mountain News*, Feb. 26, 2009, accessed at http://www.rockymountainnews.com/news/2009/feb/26/rocky-mountain-news-closes-friday-final-edition.
4. *Losing the News*, Jones, 2–3.
5. Ibid., 3–4.
6. "Newspapers Lost 105K Jobs Since 2001," Erik Sass, MediaDailyNews, Feb. 22, 2010, accessed at http://www.mediapost.com/publications/?fa=Articles.printFriendly&art_aid=122901.

7. "The Reconstruction of American Journalism," Leonard Downie and Michael Schudson, *Columbia Journalism Review*, Oct. 19, 2009, accessed at http://www.cjr.org/reconstruction/the_reconstruction_of_american.php.

8. *Losing the News*, Jones, xviii.

9. Ibid., 7.

10. U.S. Bureau of Labor Statistics, "Occupational Employment Statistics Survey," May 2008.

11. *Trust Us, We're Experts!*, John Stauber and Sheldon Rampton, Jeremy P. Tarcher/Putnam, 2001, 272.

12. *Trust Us, We're Experts!*, Stauber and Rampton, 272–74.

13. "Why Is It Taking So Long?," Brad Collins, *Solar Today*, January/February 2010, 10.

14. "Journalism 2009: Desperate Metaphors, Desperate Revenue Models, and the Desperate Need for Better Journalism," Arianna Huffington, Huffington Post, Dec. 1, 2009, http://www.huffingtonpost.com/arianna-huffington/journalism-2009-desperate_b_374642.html.

15. Ibid.

16. *Losing the News*, Jones, 8.

17. Ibid., xviii.

18. *Losing the News*, Jones, 99.

Index

A Note on the Author

Wendell Potter is the senior fellow on health care at the Center for Media and Democracy. He has appeared on countless television and radio programs and has been quoted in newspapers and magazines across the country. Prior to his twenty-five-year career in public relations, he was a journalist for the *Memphis Press-Scimitar* and Scripps Howard news service.